Le

Feeding Made Easy

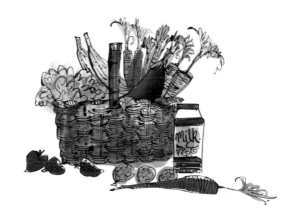

1 3 5 7 9 10 8 6 4 2

Published in 2008 by Vermilion, an imprint of Ebury Publishing

A Random House Group Company

Text copyright © Gina Ford 2008

Illustrations copyright © Mark Beech 2008

The Random House Group Limited Reg. No. 954009

Addresses for companies within the Random House Group can be found at www.randomhouse.co.uk

A CIP catalogue record for this book is available from the British Library

The Random House Group Limited supports The Forest Stewardship Council (FSC), the leading international forest certification organisation. All our titles that are printed on Greenpeace approved FSC certified paper carry the FSC logo. Our paper procurement policy can be found at www.rbooks.co.uk/environment

To buy books by your favourite authors and register for offers visit www.rbooks.co.uk

Design by Turnbull Grey
Contributions from Fiona Hinton, Registered Dietitian

Printed and bound by Firmengruppe APPL, aprinta druck, Wemding, Germany

ISBN 9780091917401

Please note that conversions to imperial weights and measures are suitable equivalents and not exact.

The information given in this book should not be treated as a substitute for qualified medical advice; always consult a medical practitioner. Neither the author nor the publisher can be held responsible for any loss or claim arising out of the use, or misuse, of the suggestions made or the failure to take medical advice.

Feeding Made Easy

From Weaning to School: the Ultimate Guide to
Contented Family Mealtimes

Gina Ford

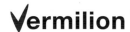
Vermilion

Contents

6   Introduction

9   Shopping Made Easy
10   Shopping
12   Organic Food
16   Fruit and Vegetables
23   Meat and Poultry
31   Fish
35   Eggs
39   Milk and Dairy
43   Grains and Pulses

51   Healthy Eating Made Easy
52   Developing Healthy Eating Habits
57   The Pitfalls of Processed Foods
61   Healthy Drinks
64   Omega-3 and Omega-6 Essential Fatty Acids
72   Antioxidants
75   Boosting the Immune System
79   Developing Appetite
81   Food Allergy and Intolerance
86   Vegetarian Children
92   Feeding During Illness

95   Mealtimes Made Easy
96   Breakfast
101   Snacks
108   Soups
111   Salads
115   Family meals
118   Food fussiness

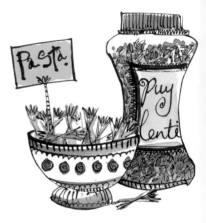

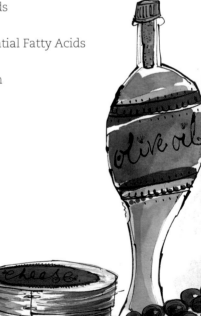

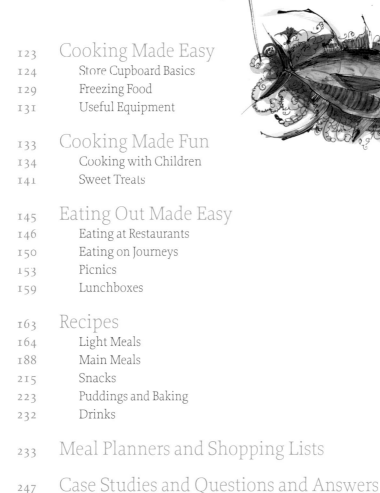

123 Cooking Made Easy
124   Store Cupboard Basics
129   Freezing Food
131   Useful Equipment

133 Cooking Made Fun
134   Cooking with Children
141   Sweet Treats

145 Eating Out Made Easy
146   Eating at Restaurants
150   Eating on Journeys
153   Picnics
159   Lunchboxes

163 Recipes
164   Light Meals
188   Main Meals
215   Snacks
223   Puddings and Baking
232   Drinks

233 Meal Planners and Shopping Lists

247 Case Studies and Questions and Answers

268 Useful Addresses

269 Index

272 Acknowledgements

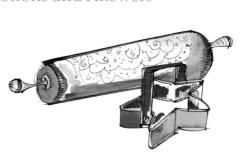

Introduction

Children need food. Parents need food. Sometimes it can feel like we spend our lives thinking about food – planning what to cook, making shopping lists, doing the weekly shop, cooking meals for the baby, the older children and then later the adults, clearing away, and of course, endlessly washing up.

While this book can't help with the washing up, I hope that it will take the pressure off some of the other areas, by providing you with weekly meal plans, shopping lists and tasty, nutritious recipes for meals which all the family can enjoy. Busy parents simply don't have time in the day to be cooking separate meals for children and adults, so these recipes are designed to appeal to all ages and to fulfill everyone's nutritional needs. Most of the recipes can be mashed or lightly puréed for the most junior members of the family, and adapted or added to for a more adult palate.

I strongly believe that one of the foundation stones of a happy life is a healthy attitude towards food and healthy eating habits. If we can get this right for our children from the outset, then they will be set for life. Of course they may go through periods of fussiness and eating less healthily, but if their early experiences of food have been positive, healthy and straightforward, then these are what will influence them and will inform their eating habits throughout life. I am constantly rewarded by witnessing the diets of the babies I have helped care for, who are now blossoming into teenagers and who continue to eat well and healthily despite the constant pressures exerted on them by the media as well as the huge presence of tantalising processed convenience foods and snacks in the shops.

This book aims to give you sensible advice and sensible recipes. In my opinion, cooking nutritious, interesting meals for the family doesn't mean that you have to offer your families five-star gourmet cooking every day nor do you have to be a great chef – in fact I know that many mums and dads don't even like cooking but are prepared to take themselves into the kitchen in order to provide good food for their families. That's the kind of food you will find here – uncomplicated, unfussy recipes that can be produced by anyone with a desire to give their children wholesome, tasty meals that will equally be enjoyed by the whole family.

The most important thing you can do, as you embark on this part of your life that involves preparing meals for your family, is RELAX. Trust your healthy, growing child to eat what he needs for continued healthy growth and to appreciate his food. Feeding should be simple – provide good food and allow your child to enjoy it. Don't allow conflict to enter the situation, with feelings of guilt, anxiety, anger or inadequacy.

Remember that children learn by imitation, so if you enjoy preparing and eating food with your family, then they will too. Contented is the mother or father who watches as the family sit together enjoying a nutritious home-cooked meal. I hope that this book will provide the tools to give you that contentment, with its advice, recipes and suggestions for healthy, happy family mealtimes.

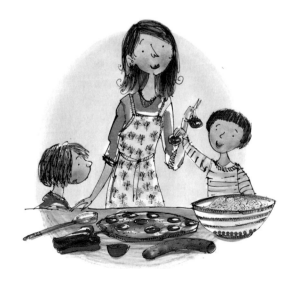

Chapter 1

Shopping
Made Easy

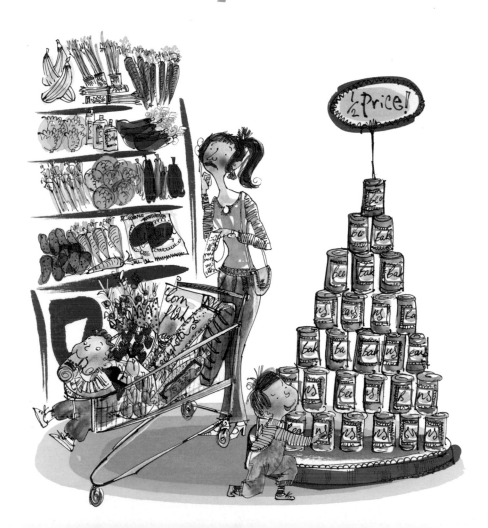

Shopping

No book about food can ignore the fact that before you can cook and eat you have to shop. With small children this can seem quite a daunting task, so find ways to make your life easier.

* Make comprehensive shopping lists so that you remember to buy everything you need, despite being distracted by your toddler in the shop.
* If shopping with small children, take healthy snacks for them to enjoy. This will prevent you having to buy expensive, highly-processed snacks which may catch their eye.
* Shop at a time of day when you know your child will be happy for a while, not when they are over-tired or hungry.
* If you have several shops you need to visit, intersperse them with a trip to a café, a quick play on the swings, or a run around the park or a friend's garden.
* Why not see if a friend with a similar-aged child is willing to do a swap? You could take it in turns to look after each other's children while you get on with an hour's shopping.
* Buy heavy and bulky items such as toilet roll and tinned and dried goods once a month, so that your weekly shop is more for the food that you need right now.
* Take advantage of local organic vegetable box deliveries, which are available all over the country. You will benefit from eating fresh, seasonal organic produce which is often locally grown, as well as avoiding carrying home heavy bags of shopping and using the car. Delivery notes often include advice on how to cook ingredients and recipes. Some schemes, such as Abel & Cole, which operates nationally, also offer delivery of a wide range of other ingredients, such as dairy produce, meat and fish.
* Try to use your local butcher, fishmonger and greengrocer. Shopping may take a little longer, but you will get more personal attention and specialist knowledge. These shops are also far more interesting for small children, who enjoy seeing rows of fish and piles of unusual fruit and vegetables. For children to develop a healthy attitude to food, it is important that they

have a respect for it and know where it comes from: the fish in their fish pie comes from a beautiful, swimming creature; carrots grow in the earth, have green feathery fronds, can be muddy and are not only available vacuum-packed and ready-chopped.

* Seek out local farmers' markets for a fun weekend family shopping experience. You may not be able to do your weekly shop at the market, but there are lots of interesting things to see and buy. Everything is local and seasonal, so you can be sure you are getting the freshest possible vegetables, fruit, meat, fish, bakery and dairy produce.

* Farm shops also give you the opportunity to buy local produce, and these frequently sell a much wider selection of goods, too. There are often animals, such as pigs and hens to look at, making it a fun trip for small children.

* Look for different shopping opportunities. Strawberry picking at a pick-your-own farm in summertime is a super activity with small children and comes with the bonus of a basket of strawberries at the end of the session. Packed with vitamin C, an essential antioxidant, strawberries are nutritious and delicious, so make the most of their seasonal appearance.

Help Your Children to Learn About Food

Visits to shops such as a greengrocer (or even the fruit and veg department of your local supermarket) can be a great opportunity for discussing with your child where the food comes from, talking about the different countries where certain fruit and vegetables grow, whether they grow under or on top of the ground or on a tree, at what time of year certain foods appear, the various colours and textures of the fruits and vegetables. Having awakened your child's curiosity, you could allow them to help you choose a new fruit or vegetable that they haven't tried before. Perhaps he could hand the money to the shopkeeper and carry his purchase himself. Children are far more likely to try something new if they have been involved in the selection of it.

Organic Food

Wherever possible, I recommend that you buy organic food for your family. Put simply, it is food which has been produced in as natural a way as possible. Conventional farming allows the use of huge amounts of artificial, chemical fertilisers and pesticides, whereas organic farming relies on predominantly natural methods to fertilise the soil and control pests. Artificial pesticides sprayed on growing crops may ensure a perfectly shaped, unblemished carrot or apple, but at what cost?

Why choose organic?

* According to a report published in the British Medical Journal, some pesticides, which cannot easily be washed off fruit and vegetables, can remain in our bodies for years, and there is concern that they may be linked to birth defects, damage to the nervous system and some cancers. By choosing organic food, you will avoid loading your child's body with such pesticides.
* Some studies indicate that organic food contains more vitamins, minerals and essential fatty acids than non-organic food. One report found that organic chickens have 25 per cent less fat than intensively-reared chickens, and free-range, organic chickens feeding on grass have higher levels of essential omega-3 fatty acids, vitamin E and beta-carotene.
* The production of organic food takes care to conserve the wildlife and environment, thereby providing a healthier world for all our children.
* I find that organic food tastes better and in some cases it is more likely to be fresher, as preservatives are not used to enhance its shelf-life.

Genetically modified food

Choosing to buy organic means that you will also be avoiding genetically modified (GM) food, as organic farming standards prohibit the use of genetically modified organisms (GMOs). Genetic modification involves manipulating the genes of plants to produce particular qualities in them. For example, one plant's resistance to drought conditions could be passed on to a more tender species to make it resistant, too. Although the effect of GMOs in food is unknown, some studies have linked their presence to adverse health effects, including allergies and disfunction of major organs such as the liver and kidneys. While the controversy over GM foods rages, the EU has introduced strict rules about labelling foods that contain GM products, and the presence of GM material or protein must be indicated on food labels.

I passionately believe that the food we eat, and especially the food we give to growing children who are more vulnerable to toxins in foods, should be as wholesome and untampered-with as possible, and that at present there is no place in our diets for GMOs – which currently appear to be more of a risk than a benefit to our health and the environment.

Is organic food worth the extra cost?

As organic farms tend to be smaller, more manageable concerns, and the additional work involved in producing organic food is more labour-intensive, organic food is frequently more expensive than the non-organic option. I do appreciate that the extra cost is a concern for families on a budget, but, in my opinion, if a choice has to be made on where to cut costs, it should not be on food. A child will not suffer from having fewer toys or more hand-me-down clothes, whereas I worry that a diet of food produced using artificial fertilisers, pesticides, antibiotics and hormones could affect his immune system and brain development for life. It is better to include organic, free-range meat and fish in your diet once or twice a week, and to make use of the vast range of readily available and economical pulses, grains, and fresh fruit and vegetables on a daily basis.

Organic for pregnant and nursing mothers

Even before the birth of your baby, it is important that you eat organically. Unborn babies can be susceptible to the toxins in a mother's body, so do try to avoid food that has been grown with the use of pesticides, as these can accumulate in a mother's body and may be passed to the growing baby. Research has also shown that breast milk can contain pesticides and that mothers who eat an organic diet have reduced levels of pesticide residues in their milk.

A non-organic apple may have been sprayed 15 times with over 30 chemicals.

Reducing pesticide intake

If it is not possible for you to eat totally organically, you can still take steps to cut down the amount of pesticides you consume.

* Thoroughly wash all fruit and vegetables.
* Peel non-organic fruit and vegetables where possible. However, even peeling doesn't remove all traces of pesticides, as bananas are heavily sprayed and still retain high levels of pesticides in the fruit beneath the skin. Do buy organic, Fair Trade bananas wherever possible.
* Grow your own. Conventionally-grown lettuce is constantly sprayed with pesticides which are difficult to wash off, and lettuce and other salad leaves are easy to grow, even in large pots. Courgettes are also fun for children, as they grow quickly and easily into large plants with bright yellow flowers; and beans (runner and French) can be made into a living, edible wigwam, climbing up bamboo sticks.
* Eat cooked vegetables instead of raw ones.
* Ensure that chicken and meat is thoroughly cooked before eating.

Recent research from America suggests that an organic diet can reduce dangerous pesticide residues in children.

If the price of organic produce restricts you, then do at least try to buy the following organic items, as research has shown that the non-organic versions contain high levels of pesticides:

* milk and dairy products
* meat and poultry
* bread
* carrots
* bananas
* lettuce
* strawberries
* ice cream

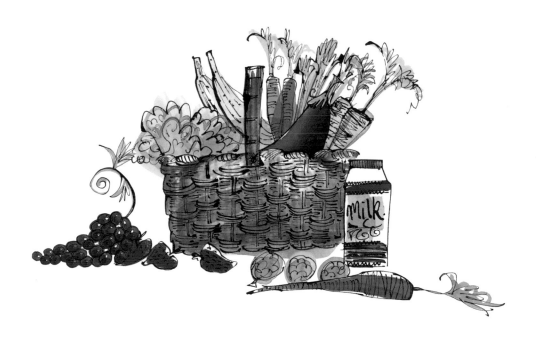

Fruit and Vegetables

To ensure a healthy diet for your family, your shopping basket should be full of fruit and vegetables. They are packed with vital vitamins, minerals and antioxidants, provide fibre and are very low in fat, so you can't do better for your child's diet than by becoming a regular at your local greengrocer or farmers' market.

Buy fresh, local, organic produce wherever possible. In buying local food you will also be purchasing the freshest seasonal fruit and vegetables, ensuring that your family benefits from a wide variety of produce and differing nutrients. In addition, buying local produce is good for the global environment as it avoids the transportation of food across the world.

What to look for when shopping

* Choose fruit and vegetables that are bright and crisp and not dull and limp, as the latter will have been on the shelves for some time.
* Carrots are sometimes sold with their feathery fronds to show how fresh they are, but do remove this greenery when you get home, to avoid goodness going out of the carrot into its leaves.
* Choose firm fruit and allow it to ripen in the fruit bowl. Very ripe fruit will bruise and spoil easily.
* Avoid potatoes which have begun to sprout.
* Go for strongly-coloured green vegetables, as any yellowing is a sign that the vegetable is spoiled.
* Buy unwaxed citrus fruit if possible.
* Always buy Fair Trade bananas.
* Ask where the produce has come from; then you can choose to buy local and British fruit and vegetables where possible.
* Ask how long the produce has been on display.

Vegetable box schemes

If you have a vegetable box delivery scheme in your area, I highly recommend that you try it. There are many benefits:

* Box schemes are a wonderful way of encouraging us all to buy the freshest, seasonal, local fruit and vegetables.
* Every week or fortnight you will receive a selection of seasonal produce delivered to your door.
* Boxes often include a recipe sheet, with suggestions on how to cook the more unusual vegetables.
* You and your child can have great fun unpacking the box, talking about the produce and discussing how you might eat the fruit and vegetables.
* You will be able to try all sorts of things that you may not have bought before, thereby broadening the range of foods in your family's diet.
* You don't have to carry heavy bags of shopping home.
* Delivery straight from the farm cuts down on lorries transporting produce to shops all over the country.

Add herbs to your shopping list

Fresh herbs start arriving in March, with parsley and mint, and continue throughout the summer. Make the most of the abundance of basil in the summer; it adds a delicious Mediterranean flavour to all sorts of salads and vegetables.

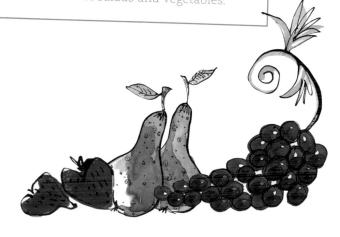

Eating with the seasons

Some vegetables, such as potatoes and onions, are stored so that they are available all year round. Other, more perishable fruit and vegetables are best enjoyed when they are in season locally. Of course, there are also delicious fruits which are not grown locally and have to be imported, such as bananas, citrus fruit, grapes, lychees, mangoes, peaches and pineapples.

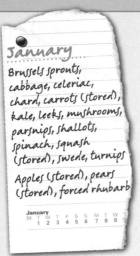

January

Brussels sprouts, cabbage, celeriac, chard, carrots (stored), kale, leeks, mushrooms, parsnips, shallots, spinach, squash (stored), swede, turnips

Apples (stored), pears (stored), forced rhubarb

January
M T W T F S S M T W T
1 2 3 4 5 6 7 8 9

February

As January, plus cauliflower, chicory and sprout tops (much under-rated – delicious and full of antioxidants)

March

Beetroot, calabrese, carrots (stored), cauliflower, kale, leeks, mushrooms, purple sprouting broccoli, radishes, spring greens

Apples (stored), pears (stored), rhubarb

July

Carrots, cauliflower, Chinese leaves, courgettes, cucumber, fennel, French beans, garlic, lettuce, mangetout, peas, peppers, salad leaves, spinach, spring onions, sweetcorn, tomatoes, watercress

Apricots, blackcurrants, blueberries, peaches, raspberries, redcurrants, strawberries

August

Carrots, cauliflower, chard, Chinese leaves, courgettes, cucumber, fennel, French beans, garlic, lettuce, mangetout, peas, peppers, runner beans, salad leaves, spinach, spring onions,

sweetcorn, tomatoes, watercress

Blackberries, greengages, peaches, plums, raspberries, strawberries

September

Beetroot, broccoli, carrots, cauliflower, chard, Chinese leaves, courgettes, cucumber, curly kale, fennel, garlic, lettuce, marrows, peas, peppers, runner beans, salad leaves, spinach, swede, sweetcorn, tomatoes, watercress

Apples, blackberries, figs, grapes, greengages, melons, pears, plums, raspberries, strawberries

By choosing local, seasonal fruit and vegetables, you will benefit from the highest nutritional value they have to offer, as vitamins are lost over time and travel. The following list shows that there is plenty to enjoy all year round – of course, this list may vary regionally and according to how successful the harvest has been.

April

Carrots (stored), kale, leeks, lettuce, mushrooms, purple sprouting broccoli, radishes, spinach, spring cabbage, watercress, wild garlic

Apples (stored), pears (stored), rhubarb

May

Asparagus, broad beans, cabbage, new carrots, cauliflower, leeks, lettuce, mushrooms, new potatoes, spinach, spring onions, watercress

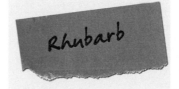

Rhubarb

June

Asparagus, aubergines, broad beans, carrots, cauliflower, Chinese leaves, courgettes, fennel, green beans, lettuce, mangetout, peas, peppers, spinach, spring onions, tomatoes, watercress

Apricots, cherries, gooseberries, peaches, raspberries, redcurrants, rhubarb, strawberries

October

Beetroot, Brussels sprouts, courgettes, kale, mushrooms, pumpkin, squash

Apples, pears, quince

November

Brussels sprouts, cabbage – Savoy and red, celeriac, celery, leeks, mushrooms, parsnips, pumpkin, squash, swede

Apples, pears, quince

December

Brussels sprouts, cabbage – Savoy and red, celeriac, celery, chard, leeks, mushrooms, parsnips, pumpkin, spinach, squash, swede, turnip

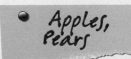

Apples, Pears

Five-a-day

There is growing evidence to show that people who eat plenty of fruit and vegetables are less likely to develop heart disease and some cancers in later life.

The current government guidelines are that we should all eat at least five portions of fruit or vegetables a day. Aim to include more than this amount in your family's diet and you will be giving them the healthiest and most delicious meals and snacks.

There are many ways to include fruit and vegetables in your diet, but it is useful to know what constitutes a portion. The table below is suitable for children over the age of six. Portion sizes for children aged between one and six should be about half of those indicated – although the quantity of fruit juice remains the same. You can enjoy fruit and vegetables which are fresh, frozen, tinned or dried to make up your five portions a day. Do try to include as much fresh produce as possible – this generally has the highest proportion of vitamins.

One portion = 80 g (3 oz) = any of the following items

* 1 apple, banana, pear, orange or other similar sized fruit
* 2 plums or similar sized fruit
* ½ a grapefruit or avocado
* 1 slice of large fruit, such as melon or pineapple
* 3 heaped tablespoons of vegetables
  (raw, cooked, frozen or tinned)
* 3 heaped tablespoons of beans and pulses (however
  much you eat, beans and pulses count as a maximum
  of one portion a day)
* 3 heaped tablespoons of fruit salad
  (fresh or tinned in fruit juice) or stewed fruit
* 1 heaped tablespoon of dried fruit (such as raisins and apricots)
* 1 handful of grapes, cherries or berries
* a dessert bowl of salad
* a glass (150 ml/5 fl oz) of fruit juice (however much you drink,
  fruit juice counts as a maximum of one portion a day)

Source: Food Standards Agency

Easy ways to include fruit and vegetables in your diet

* Drink a glass of fresh, pure fruit juice with meals. This can count as one portion.
* Make fruit smoothies with a mixture of fresh fruit (see page 104).
* Add a handful of dried fruit to porridge or breakfast cereal.
* Top breakfast toast with sliced banana.
* Include a side salad with your main meal.
* Make a large bowl of fruit salad and keep, covered in the fridge, for the family to enjoy whenever they need a snack.
* Make ice lollies from pure fruit juice or freeze fruit smoothies for a healthy summer treat.
* Add vegetables to pasta sauces.
* Always include salad in sandwiches.
* Always include fresh fruit in lunchboxes.
* Have a large bowl of fresh, washed fruit on the table and encourage the family to choose snacks from it.
* Make sorbets and ice cream from fresh fruit.
* Use puréed vegetables to thicken sauces or for tasty dips.
* A serving of pulses (beans, lentils, etc.) counts as one portion of fruit and vegetables.
* Snack on a handful of dried fruit or a piece of fresh fruit.
* Keep a selection of prepared vegetable sticks in a box in the fridge and offer with dips for a delicious snack.
* Add fruit to jelly, as a treat, to encourage children to enjoy fruit. Try satsumas, apricots, plums, bananas, grapes, berries, cherries (stoned) or tinned fruit in natural juice.
* If your child doesn't like the taste of cooked cabbage, try offering him a salad of finely sliced white cabbage mixed with grated carrot, some natural yoghurt and a handful of raisins.

Getting the most out of your fruit and vegetables

To get the maximum benefit from the vitamins and minerals in fruit and vegetables:

* Buy and eat them as fresh as possible.
* Use frozen vegetables which have been frozen immediately after picking to conserve vitamins.
* Steam or lightly cook vegetables as over-cooking most vegetables reduces their vitamin content.
* Don't cut fruit and vegetables until you are ready to use them.
* Don't allow cut fruit and vegetables to sit, soaking in water, as the vitamins will disappear into the water.
* Use the vegetable cooking water to make soups, stocks and gravy, as this will contain vitamins lost from the vegetables.
* Serve fruit and vegetables rich in vitamin C, such as citrus fruit and peppers, or a glass of pure orange juice, with iron-rich vegetables such as spinach, as the vitamin C improves the iron absorption.
* Eat a wide variety of fruit and vegetables to give you the complete range of nutrients.

Parsley – more than just a garnish

Fresh parsley is a great source of vitamin C, though you'll need to eat plenty of it to really reap the benefits. Add finely chopped fresh parsley to all kinds of vegetables, such as carrots, courgettes, potatoes, sweet potatoes, squash and sweetcorn. If children are always presented with these dishes flecked with green then they are less likely to develop a dislike for meals with 'green things' in.

Meat and Poultry

Meat is one of the best ways of including first-class protein in your child's diet. However, the supermarket aisles are full of packets of meat in a mesmerising array of cuts, and it can be difficult to know what to buy.

In your search for good quality meat for your family, my first recommendation is to make friends with a butcher. If you are lucky enough to live near a butcher's shop, then use it. You can tell by the look of the meat on display, and the state of the shop itself, whether this is a place you wish to frequent. Start talking to your butcher and ask his advice. He is likely to be extremely knowledgeable and helpful about the meat he sells, and will be able to suggest cuts of meat to suit your needs and your purse. There is far more available than lamb chops and minced beef, so go in and have a look – and try different things.

Taking your child with you is a good way of establishing a healthy respect for food. If we are going to eat meat, then I believe we should acknowledge and understand where it came from. Children should not grow up thinking that chicken drumsticks come from a polystyrene packet in the supermarket. Giving your child an awareness of meat and its origins is an essential part of his education concerning food.

Some local butchers takes in parties of primary school children to show them how to make sausages. Why not see if your local butcher might do this? The children are then able to eat what they have made – and will learn to appreciate the best handmade, meat-rich sausages.

When shopping for meat, it is worth remembering:

* The meat you buy should be farm-reared and local where possible.
* Any animal that has led as natural a life as is feasible, enjoying a free-range existence, and with a natural diet, will produce meat of far greater quality than that from intensively reared animals.
* To increase production of milk and meat, intensively farmed cattle are fed on grain rather than grass, and this affects the quality of the meat.
* Some research suggests that the meat and milk from cattle which are allowed to graze naturally on grass has a higher proportion of the essential omega-3 oils than that from intensively reared animals.
* Organically reared animals are raised in a humane manner, which many people believe will improve the quality of the meat they produce.
* Organic meat comes from animals fed on a natural diet of foods free from pesticides, hormones and antibiotics, so by buying organic meat, you avoid any concern about harmful residues which may be present in non-organic meat. As I've already mentioned, this is of particular importance for children, whose systems are more vulnerable.

I really believe that it is better to buy a small quantity of organic or free-range meat and chicken and enjoy it as a family treat, once or twice a week, than to serve poorer quality, intensively produced meat more often.

Remember that good quality meat will go further, as there will be less fat and water added.

Top tip

Buy a chicken and serve as a roast. You should have enough left over for another meal and some sandwiches, as well as being able to make delicious stock from the bones, with which you can make tempting soups and risottos.

The next question is: what cuts of meat do you need and how should you cook them?

Beef

* The general rule with beef is that the more expensive, leaner cuts come from the rear of the animal. (The cattle's hind legs are the ones most employed in movement, so there is less fat on the meat from these quarters.)
* The leaner cuts are suitable for roasting, starting with the top-quality sirloin, which is ideal for a family celebration.
* The topsides – top rump, topside, silverside and aitch-bone are half the price of sirloin and make great family joints for roasting.
* For a real treat, choose prime-quality fillet steak, which is extremely tender and quick and easy to cook.
* Rump steak is great for stir fries as it is also tender and cooks quickly.
* Use topsides for a wonderful pot-roast as they won't dry out and will impart a wonderful flavour to any vegetables cooked alongside.
* Roasting joints should be roasted for about 15 – 20 minutes per 450 g (1 lb).
* If you have the option of a fan or conventional oven, use the conventional one, as fan ovens can dry out roasting joints.
* Overcooked beef can become dry, so keep an eye on it towards the end of the cooking time.
* It is important to have a certain amount of fat in beef to impart flavour and retain moisture, so some leaner cuts may be sold with an extra layer of fat attached. Don't discard this, but cook the joint as it is sold.
* If you are making gravy to serve with your roast beef, retain the cooking juices in the roasting tin. With the addition of some stock or the water used to cook vegetables, you have the makings of delicious gravy.
* The front half of the animal provides the stewing meats, which may be displayed as chuck steak, blade, brisket or stewing joints.
* Brisket also makes a tasty pot-roast – cooked with seasonal root vegetables for a one-pot meal.
* Minced beef is usually made from the stewing meats, as a little fat is necessary to prevent toughness.

* Lean minced beef has less fat, but unscrupulous butchers may just put it through the mincer again, as this makes the fat disappear into the meat.
* Stews and casseroles take time to cook but require very little effort and are extremely tasty. Ask your butcher for advice if you are unsure how long to cook the meat. The longer you cook it, the more tender it will be.
* When buying meat for a casserole, allow about 100–150 g (4–6 oz) per adult. You will need about the same amount of minced beef as stewing beef.
* When buying beef, look for meat which is red or purplish, as a brown colour indicates that the beef has been sitting out in the air for too long and has spoiled. The fat should be white in colour, not yellow.

When serving roast meats, don't forget the accompaniments – chutneys, fruit jellies and sauces. They are a great way of introducing a variety of new flavours which will enhance the taste of the meat without the need for salt. Offer your child a taste – you might be surprised at the sophistication of his palate.

Lamb

* The most common roasting joint is the leg, which is ideal for a simple roast and is quite lean if trimmed. This comes from the back of the animal.
* The front leg forms the shoulder, which is slightly fatter but I find it has a better flavour.
* The shoulder is cheaper than the leg and very versatile as it can be used for a pot roast (traditionally with white beans), or boned, rolled and stuffed.
* Shoulder of lamb can also be used cubed, for curries and casseroles.
* For a summer barbecue, ask your butcher for a butterflied leg of lamb. This is boned out and flattened, and quick to cook.
* The centre part of the lamb produces a variety of chops: chump, which are the most expensive; loin, which are top quality; and cutlets, which are great for everyday grills. All of these can be successfully barbecued as well as grilled.
* Lamb shanks are increasingly popular and are wonderful cooked slowly for several hours. Serve one per adult.
* Neck of lamb is excellent for stews and hotpots.

* Lamb can be a fatty meat and the fat in stews may need draining and skimming, although recent improved breeding has reduced the amount of fat in some cases.
* Lean lamb, cooked and served with all visible fat removed, is a low-fat meat.
* Choose lamb which is firm and pink, with a fine texture. Any fat on the meat should be white, not yellow.
* Roasting joints should be roasted for about 20 minutes per 450 g (1 lb), plus another 20 minutes.

Top tip

Lamb is traditionally served with mint sauce, but for a healthy new take on this, which may be more appealing to children, mix fresh chopped mint leaves with natural yoghurt and maybe some finely chopped garlic.

Pork

* There is an old butcher's saying that you can eat every part of a pig but its squeak, and it certainly is a universally enjoyed and versatile meat.
* Pork can be intensively farmed, so always look for outdoor-reared or organic pork. It is worth paying slightly more for your pork, knowing that the pigs have led a natural life, fed on a mixed diet and been allowed to forage for food.
* By buying your pork at a farmers' market, you can be sure that the meat is raised locally, and usually produced without the use of any artificial additives or preservatives.
* Every joint of pork is suitable for roasting as it is all so tender.
* A whole leg of pork, sometimes called a fresh ham, is a superb choice for a large party. For smaller celebrations, choose a half-leg.
* There is sometimes confusion over the difference between gammon and ham, but they are in fact the same thing. Gammon generally sold uncooked, however, while ham is usually sold cooked.
* Shoulder of pork, either on the bone or boned and rolled, makes an excellent, economical roast.

- For pot roasts and braises, choose shoulder, chump chops, leg steaks or belly of pork.
- Pork fillet is extra lean, and is ideal for stir fries as well as casseroles.
- Pork loin makes a lean and tasty roasting joint, which is easy to cook and serve. It is also great for stir fries.
- For grilling and barbecuing, choose pork chops, belly slices or leg steaks.
- Bacon, either green (unsmoked) or smoked, is cured pork, which has been preserved in salt. Do remember that bacon is extremely salty and should not be given to children under the age of 18 months. Enjoy bacon in small quantities, mixed with other foods and no added salt, or as a weekend treat.
- Buy sausages from your local butcher to ensure that you are getting the healthiest option. Butchers' sausages must contain 65 per cent meat by law, but try to buy ones which are 85 per cent pork. A certain amount of fat is needed to produce a succulent sausage, and the ideal ratio is 85 per cent meat to 15 per cent fat. Sausages should only contain meat, such as belly, knuckle and shoulder trim, mixed with a wheat and milk rusk to bind. Salt levels are also governed by law. There may be spices, herbs, or even fruit and vegetables such as apple and leek for additional flavour. If you have a wheat allergy and are concerned about gluten, your butcher may be able to make gluten-free sausages for you. Most butchers' sausages are made with natural casings.
- Chipolatas are thinner sausages with a thinner casing. They are a popular choice for children as they are quicker to cook and a convenient size.
- Roast pork for about 20 minutes per 450 g (1 lb), plus another 20 minutes.
- Traditionally, apple sauce is served with roast pork, and many children like this combination of sweet and savoury.

Chicken and turkey

- Organic chickens are those raised in a more natural habitat without the use of hormones and antibiotics.
- Free-range birds are allowed access to the outdoors. Ensure that any free-range chicken or eggs you buy are truly from birds which have been allowed to roam outside over a large area.
- A healthy, natural environment, a mixed diet, and the freedom to range

and forage will produce the best-tasting chicken.

* Factory-farmed chickens contain more fat and less iron than traditional breeds of chicken, which are raised in humane, organic or free-range environments.
* Chicken and turkey are very low-fat meats, once the skin is removed. (The skin can double the amount of fat.)
* The dark meat is higher in fat than the light meat, such as the breast.
* As well as whole chicken, choose quarters, thighs, drumsticks and wings, which are all ideal for roasting, and for casseroles.
* Look for birds which smell fresh, are firm to the touch, with an opaque skin. The skin colour can vary – it may be yellow if the chicken is corn-fed.
* Your butcher will be happy to joint a chicken for you if you need chicken pieces for your recipe.
* Boneless chicken breasts are low in fat and quick to cook, but can become dry. Use for stir fries, risottos or pasta dishes.
* For the tastiest roast chicken, roast the bird breast down. This keeps the breast moist and juicy during the additional time needed to cook the dark meat until tender.
* Poultry can contain low levels of salmonella and campylobacter – the bacteria which can lead to food poisoning if they multiply – so raw chicken must be handled and stored hygienically. Always refrigerate as soon as possible after purchase. If giblets are present, remove them and store separately.
* Roast chicken and turkey for about 20 minutes per 450 g (1 lb), plus another 20 minutes.
* Always ensure poultry is cooked thoroughly. To test a whole roast bird, pierce the thickest part of the thigh with a skewer. Only when the juices run clear – not at all pink – is the poultry cooked.

Liver

Liver is a good choice for families as it is highly nutritious, quick to cook and economical. It is a good source of protein and contains vitamins A, B and D, and iron. Choose lamb's liver, which is dark-coloured and smells fresh. Calf's liver is a delicious, highly-prized treat. Pig's liver has a stronger flavour. To cook liver, simmer in water until tender or pan fry. Note that infants and young children should not eat liver or liver products more than once a week. and pregnant women should avoid them as they may take in too much vitamin A.

Rabbit

Rabbit is very low in fat and cholesterol, so is a good healthy and economical choice. It has a slightly stronger flavour than chicken but is delicious in slow-cooked casseroles. Ensure you add plenty of liquid during cooking to retain moisture. Tame rabbit will be plumper and have a more delicate flavour than the stronger taste of wild rabbit.

Things to remember once you get your meat home

* Always store raw meat in the fridge, away from cooked foods.
* Don't allow juices from raw meat to drip onto other foods in the fridge.
* Don't put cooked meat on the same plate that has had raw meat.
* If you are marinating meat, don't add uncooked marinade to cooked beef, as it contains raw juices which may contain bacteria.
* Always wash utensils that have touched raw meat, before using them for cooked meat.
* Don't partially cook meat, refrigerate, and finish cooking at a later time, as this allows bacteria to develop.
* Store leftover meat and poultry in the fridge as soon as it is cold. Never refrigerate warm meat.
* Consume leftover meat and poultry within two to three days.

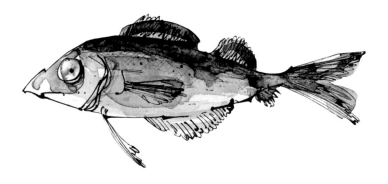

Fish

For a source of first-class protein, it is hard to beat fish. In addition to being a fantastic source of protein, fish also provides vitamins, minerals such as selenium and iodine, and is low in saturated fat.

Oily fish is a superb source of omega-3 fatty acids. Fish is easily digested, quick to cook and highly versatile, and it is recommended that we should eat at least two portions of it a week, including one portion of oily fish. Because fish is low in saturated fat, I recommend that you use it as much as possible in your family's diet in place of meat, which, although a similarly good source of protein, often has a much higher fat content.

Getting the best

There is a dizzying array of fish available at fishmongers and supermarkets, but it is all too easy to buy the familiar favourites – cod, haddock and tuna. Unfortunately their popularity has led to dangerously low stock levels.

* There are a lot of delicious, alternative and undervalued species of fish, so ask your fishmonger to recommend something different.
* Look for organically and sustainably-farmed fish.
* To ensure that your fish comes from a sustainable source, shop where you see the Marine Stewardship Council logo, as this will guarantee sustainability.
* Question your fishmonger about where his fish comes from and how it was caught.
* Try to buy line-caught fish, as drift-net fishing can damage the sea bed and harm other marine life.
* Buy locally caught fish when available – this will be fresher and has not been air-freighted on ice.
* Intensive fish-farming methods can lead to overcrowding and the proliferation of disease. When buying farmed fish, choose those farmed in open-sea conditions to avoid buying contaminated fish.

What to look for when buying fish

* As it is highly perishable it is vital to buy fish that is spankingly fresh.
* Always buy from somewhere that receives daily supplies of fish.
* Buy fish that is refrigerated or on ice.
* Don't buy frozen fish or shellfish which has damaged packaging.
* Choose fish with clear, bright, glassy, slightly bulging eyes.
* Fish should have moist, bright skin, firm to the touch. Scales should be shiny and there should be none missing.
* Fresh fish should smell clean and sea-like, not strongly fishy.
* When buying smoked fish, choose undyed varieties, without added colour.
* Buy prawns which are dry, bright and firm.
* Buy fish at the end of your shopping trip, and take it straight home to refrigerate.

Choosing fish

Different types of fish are suitable for a variety of cooking methods, so choose your fish according to your recipe. Be flexible – only buy fish which is fresh and change your menu plans if necessary. However, fish is extremely versatile and different species can often be substituted for one another in recipes.

For making fish pies and stews, choose loins or fillets of chunky white fish such as haddock, smoked fish, salmon and prawns.

For grilling and pan frying, choose thin fillets of flat fish such as plaice. Cook with skin on to retain moisture.

For kebabs, choose chunks of firm, meaty fish such as monkfish or tuna.

For baking, choose thick fillets, loins or steaks, or whole fish such as mackerel, snapper, sea bass and salmon.

Shellfish, such as prawns, mussels, crab, lobster, squid and scallops, are low in fat, high in protein and an excellent source of minerals, such as selenium, zinc, copper and iodine. However, due to the risk of allergy and food poisoning, I recommend you avoid shellfish until your child is 18 months old.

Avoid shark, swordfish and marlin for children under the age of sixteen, as they can contain high levels of mercury which may damage a child's developing nervous system (see additional precautions on page 69).

When you get your fish home

* Put fish and shellfish in the fridge or freezer as soon as you get home, making sure that they are wrapped or covered.
* Don't allow raw fish or shellfish to come into contact with cooked foods.
* If marinating seafood, place in the fridge. If you want to use the uncooked marinade to serve with the fish, put some aside before using to marinate the raw fish.
* Wash your hands before handling raw fish or shellfish.
* Use separate utensils for preparing raw fish or shellfish.
* Thaw frozen fish or shellfish in the fridge.

Top tip

* Ask your fishmonger to scale, clean and fillet your fish if necessary.
* Fish cooked on the bone has a better flavour, so cook fish unboned if possible, and the flesh will fall from the bone easily once cooked.
* Always remove all bones from fish served to children to avoid choking.

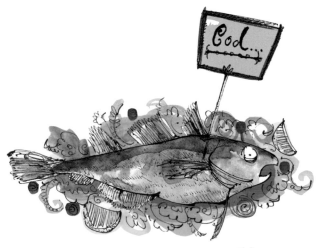

Canned fish

Canned fish is both convenient and healthy. The canning process ensures that the bones are soft, and may be eaten, providing an excellent source of calcium.

Canned tuna is a nutritious choice but it doesn't contain the levels of omega-3 fatty acids which are present in fresh tuna.

Canned sardines–lightly mashed–make a great sandwich filling, or try mackerel and pilchards on toast for a tasty and healthy snack.

Canned red salmon is usually wild, so is a great option if you are trying to avoid buying farmed fish.

Recipes using fish:

Linguine with Tuna and Tomato (page 188)
Mild Salmon and Coconut Curry (page 190)
Fish and Prawn Pie with Crunchy Oat Topping (page 197)
Baked Fish with Quinoa and Roasted Tomatoes (page 213)
Salad Niçoise (page 208)
Pasta with Salmon and Broccoli (page 214)
Gently Spiced Monkfish (page 201)
Prawn Risotto (page 211)
Favourite Fishcakes (page 176)

Eggs

Eggs are one of the greatest convenience foods. If you have a box of eggs in the kitchen you can create a delicious, nutritious meal in minutes.

Nutritionally, eggs are a valuable part of a healthy diet. They are an excellent source of protein, containing all the essential amino acids needed by the body. In addition, they provide many of the minerals needed by the body, including zinc, phosphorous, selenium, iodine and iron, and are also a significant source of several B vitamins as well as containing vitamins A and D. On top of this, they have a relatively low saturated fat content. In the past it was thought that we should limit consumption of eggs, due to their high cholesterol content, but recent research has shown that it is largely saturated fats which contribute to raised cholesterol levels, so eggs will only have a minor effect on the level of cholesterol in the body. So if you and your family enjoy a healthy balanced diet, make space in it for eggs.

Buying eggs

Choose organic eggs where possible. They do cost more, as organic chickens require more land and more work, but in buying certified organic eggs you can be sure that the chickens that laid them are fed a natural diet without the inclusion of pesticides, hormones or antibiotics, and are allowed to roost and forage in a happy environment. Free-range eggs are the next best choice, as these chickens are kept in much better conditions than battery ones and are free to roam. However, some free-range birds are free-range in name only, as they are kept in barns, with only a small opening providing access to the outside, which is often blocked by other birds. To be certain that your eggs are truly free-range, try to buy local ones from small farms or farmers' markets, and ask the seller about the size of the flock of chickens. Large flocks of over 2,000 chickens in one barn may experience lower welfare than those in smaller flocks. Eggs from battery hens are considerably cheaper than free-range or organic eggs, but at a high price to the chickens, which are kept in appalling, unnatural conditions, confined in small cages with very little space to move around. As a consequence, the eggs they lay are often watery and pale, and inferior to the rich, dense eggs laid by happier hens.

Egg safety

* Because of the slight risk of the salmonella bacteria being present in raw eggs, I recommended that you do not introduce whole eggs into your child's diet until he is at least nine months old.
* Some foods contain raw egg, and these should not be given to very young children, whose immune systems are still developing, or to pregnant women or the elderly. Foods which may contain raw egg include homemade mayonnaise or ice cream, hollandaise sauce, some salad dressings, icing and certain desserts such as tiramisu and mousse.
* Eggs can cause an allergic reaction, so if there is a history of allergy in the family then it is advisable to wait until your child is one year old before you offer him eggs.
* Do not give your young child lightly cooked eggs.
* Don't use eggs with cracked or damaged shells, as dirt or bacteria may have entered the egg.
* Eggs should be stored in a cool place, away from strong-smelling foods.
* To test an egg for freshness, place it in a bowl of water—if it floats to the surface it is likely to be old and possibly bad (because the size of the natural air pocket in the egg increases with age). If the egg sinks to the bottom, it is fresh.
* Look for the date-stamped mark on egg shells, and do not keep eggs longer than the best-before date specified.

Versatile eggs

Once your child can enjoy eggs, there is no end to the possibilities for quick and easy meals that eggs can provide.

* A simple boiled egg with fingers of buttered wholemeal toast makes a comforting tea. More adventurous children and adults might also like some lightly steamed asparagus spears, in season, to dip in their egg.
* Scrambled eggs are good partners with lots of foods, their delicate flavour marrying well with vegetables such as tomatoes and mushrooms, as well as contrasting with the gutsy flavours of smoked fish, olives and tangy cheeses. Try smoked mackerel—an easily-available and tasty oily

fish, rich in omega-3. Pile the lightly scrambled egg mixed with flakes of smoked mackerel onto toasted buttered muffins or granary toast. With the addition of some grilled, halved tomatoes, or cherry tomatoes and chunks of cucumber, you have a light lunch or tea.

* When your child's tastes become more adventurous, serve scrambled eggs 'Ranch Style', with sautéed onions, peppers, garlic and coriander, wrapped in soft tortillas, or Mexican style, with a spicy tomato sauce, chopped avocado and coriander.

* Scrambled eggs and smoked salmon is a classic and sumptuous combination, and makes a treat for a weekend breakfast or brunch for the whole family – particularly good for nursing mothers for whom good nutrition is essential to ensure that their milk supply is maintained, as well as ensuring that the mother has enough energy to cope with demands made by the rest of the family. For a family with a toddler and a new baby, a delicious weekend brunch together goes a long way to building happy family dynamics, giving the toddler a chance to eat in a relaxed environment with both Mum and Dad, who are able to focus totally on him, perhaps at a time when the new baby isn't around.

* Omelettes can be enjoyed plain or packed with all kinds of additions – grated cheese, ham, chopped fresh herbs, grilled mushrooms, lightly cooked vegetables such as peppers, courgettes, spinach, sweetcorn or even peas.

* For a more substantial meal, add eggs to sautéed onions and potatoes to make a Spanish omelette, or make a frittata with courgettes and cheese. These are equally delicious cold and make ideal finger food, cut into chunks, for toddlers. (See page 167.) You can also pack slices or chunks in lunchboxes, or take them on picnics with a pot of homemade tomato sauce as a dip.

* Hard-boiled eggs also make great picnic food. Transport in their shells and serve peeled and quartered, or mash with a little butter for a nutritious sandwich filling, along with chopped tomato or cress. Alternatively, take slices of hard-boiled egg, avocado, finely chopped tomato and chopped fresh coriander and serve in wraps or wholemeal bread.

* To make an eggy dip, mash hard-boiled egg with a little mayonnaise and Greek yoghurt and add finely chopped watercress. Serve with breadsticks,

rye sticks, savoury crackers or vegetable chunks.

* Poached eggs make a nourishing light meal served on a bed of chopped, steamed spinach, or piled onto muffins or crumpets with ham and topped with cheese sauce.

* For an instant snack, dip slices of bread into beaten egg and fry in butter to make eggy bread (see page 169). Cut into fingers and serve with homemade tomato sauce. For a breakfast treat, you can dip fruit bread into egg with a pinch of cinnamon added, before frying.

* Eggs are an essential ingredient in pancakes (see page 215). Make large ones and serve them wrapped around scrambled egg and smoked fish, tuna with a tomato sauce, or chopped chicken in a white sauce. Plain pancakes can be batch cooked and frozen with a layer of greaseproof paper between each layer – ready to be defrosted when you need a quick meal.

* Scotch pancakes make a tasty breakfast, served with natural yoghurt and chopped fresh fruit, or American-style with crispy bacon and maple syrup for a substantial brunch. (Use the recipe for energy-packed Oaty Breakfast Pancakes on page 215.)

* For a simple supper, make egg-fried rice with peas (see page 179), or toss cooked egg noodles and steamed green beans in a little light soy sauce and a dash of sesame oil, and serve topped with a thin omelette, rolled up and sliced.

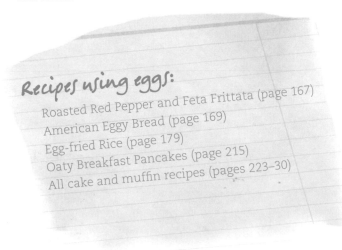

Recipes using eggs:
Roasted Red Pepper and Feta Frittata (page 167)
American Eggy Bread (page 169)
Egg-fried Rice (page 179)
Oaty Breakfast Pancakes (page 215)
All cake and muffin recipes (pages 223–30)

Milk and Dairy

Milk and dairy products are great sources of protein and vitamins A, B12 and D, as well as being principal sources of easily-absorbed calcium.

Between the ages of one and six, it is important that your child gets enough calcium to build strong bones and teeth. This is easy to achieve if he is given sufficient quantities of milk or equivalent dairy products. The daily recommendation for one- to two-year-olds is 500 ml (17 fl oz) of milk, with 350 ml (12 fl oz) being the minimum requirement. Children over the age of two should have a maximum of 350 ml of milk. However, in addition to milk, this total can be made up of other dairy products, such as yoghurt and cheese. A 125 g (4 ½ oz) pot of yoghurt is equivalent to 210 ml (about 7 fl oz) of milk, as is 30 g (1 oz) of cheese – which is a piece about the size of a matchbox. So, if your toddler has a large cup of milk in his porridge, on his breakfast cereal or to drink, and then later has a yoghurt and maybe a little cheese, he is easily meeting the recommendation.

Up to the age of two it is important that you give your child whole or full-fat milk, as the fat is essential for healthy growth. After the age of two, you may give him semi-skimmed milk.

Organic milk for health

Recent research has shown that organic milk has all the nutritional goodness of non-organic milk but, due to the cows' more natural diet, it also has the following additional health benefits:

Essential vitamins and minerals Omega-3 is an essential fatty acid and is vital for good health, playing a part in maintaining heart health, amongst other benefits. Studies have confirmed that organic milk naturally contains much more omega-3 than non-organic milk. This is thought to be due to the fact that organic cows are fed higher levels of natural red clover than non-organic cows. Organic milk can contain up to 71 per cent more omega-3 than non-organic milk and has a better ratio of omega-3 to omega-6. Research has also established that organic milk has higher levels of vitamin E, which protects the body's cells; vitamin A, important for vision and development; and other antioxidants, which help prevent cancer.

No unwanted additives As well as having clear health benefits, drinking organic milk also minimises the risk of consuming chemical residues. Some experts believe children may be particularly susceptible to pesticide residues as they have a higher intake of food per unit of body weight than adults, have immature organ systems, and may have limited ability to detoxify these substances. The British Society for Ecological Medicine also believes there is good evidence linking the rise in incidence of allergies with a general over-exposure to chemicals including pesticides. Organic milk is produced in a natural way, which means that the cows do not graze on pastures sprayed with artificial, chemical pesticides, are not fed GM cattle feed and are only ever treated with antibiotics when they are actually ill.

Yoghurt

This is a great source of body-building protein and calcium, and is generally popular with children. Nowadays much of the natural yoghurt available is 'live' yoghurt. This contains beneficial bacteria cultures which many people believe help digestion as well as boosting the immune system. All yoghurt contains the bacteria *Lactobacillus bulgaricus* and *Streptococcus thermophilus*, and 'bio' or 'live' yoghurt also contains one or more of *Lactobacillus acidophilus*, *bifidobacterium* and *Lactobacillus casei*.

For children under the age of five, choose natural yoghurt made from whole milk. Low-fat varieties are not suitable as young children need the fat to grow – and in fact there is not a lot of fat in any natural yoghurt.

There is a wide range of yoghurts targeted specifically at children. These are very convenient as they come in small pots and tubes, but I recommend that they are only used occasionally as they can contain high levels of sugar, artificial sweeteners and flavouring. If you do buy fruit yoghurts, look for those containing real fruit purée. Spend a little while reading the labels and get to know which yoghurts are the most natural. Don't be swayed by your child's requests for the ones with the latest television or Disney characters on the packet.

Buy large pots of natural yoghurt and serve topped with homemade fruit purée (see page 143), a drizzle of honey or a spoonful of pure fruit spread.

Greek yoghurt has a thick, creamy texture. It can be a delicious and a healthier alternative to ice cream or cream with many desserts, and also works well as a substitute for cream in cooking. Traditionally made from sheep's milk, many 'Greek style' yoghurts are now made from cow's milk.

You can use plain, natural yoghurt to replace mayonnaise in potato, chicken and tuna salads, and in coleslaw.

Cheese

* Cheese is a good source of calcium, but can also be high in fat. Lower-fat cheeses to try include cottage cheese, curd cheese (also called fromage frais), Edam and mozzarella.
* Feta cheese is lower in fat but soaked in brine, and so is extremely salty. To remove the saltiness, soak it in water or milk for half an hour before use.
* When using cheese to flavour a sauce, choose a strong cheese such as mature Cheddar, as you will need to use less.
* For snacks and sandwiches, mild Cheddar is more suitable for children's palates.
* Look for regional British cheeses to extend your child's range. Red Leicester and Double Gloucester are popular with children, but others to try include Wensleydale, Lancashire and Cheshire, which have a drier, crumbly texture.
* Offer children a little cheese with some grapes or slices of apple as a dessert, to develop their savoury rather than their sweet palate.

Recipes using dairy products:

Tagliatelle with Lemon and Courgette Sauce (page 191)
Creamy Vegetarian Lasagne (page 200)
The Best Macaroni Cheese (page 207)
Green Monster Pasta (page 173)
Pizza (page 182)
Sweetcorn Chowder (page 186)
Mini Courgette Rosti Cakes (page 185)
Oaty Breakfast Pancakes (page 215)
Homemade Pesto sauce (page 184)
Courgette Cornmeal Muffins (page 216)
Strawberry Yoghurt Ice Cream (page 224)

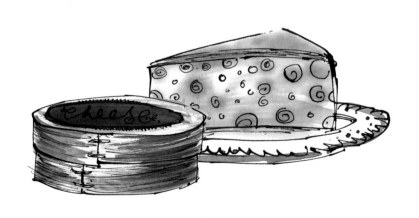

Grains and Pulses

During my time working with families in the Middle East and Asia, I was introduced to the wonderful versatility and nutritional value of grains and pulses. Across the world, these have traditionally been used much more widely than in Britain, and I am delighted that there is a fast-growing awareness and appreciation of these foods in the West.

Research suggests that eating grains and pulses is beneficial to health. They are a useful source of dietary fibre, both insoluble (found in wholemeal bread, brown rice, and wholegrain cereals as well as in fruit and vegetables) – to prevent bowel disorders, constipation and protect against colon cancer – and soluble (found in oats and pulses) – thought to reduce cholesterol.

Recommendations for healthy eating suggest incorporating more fibre in our diets, and this is easily achievable if you take advantage of the widespread availability and affordability of grains and pulses. As they are grown and used all over the world, you will discover different grains and pulses included in recipes from across the globe. It is hard to imagine an Indian curry without rice, a Middle Eastern mezze without hummus made from chickpeas, or a French cassoulet without haricot beans.

Grains and pulses are also great convenience foods. Dried and ready-packed, they can be kept for up to a year, stored away from light, in a dry, airtight container. However, pulses do toughen as they get older and will take longer to cook, so it is advisable to eat them as fresh as possible. Tinned pulses are extremely convenient and easy to use as they require no soaking and are already cooked. Check that they don't have high levels of added sugar or salt. Once drained and rinsed they are ideal for adding to soups, stews and salads, or puréeing into tasty dips.

Small children and high-fibre diets

Wholegrain cereals and high-fibre food should not be served exclusively to small children. Children under five have small tummies and high energy needs, and these foods may fill them up without providing sufficient nutrition. Balance these foods with more refined cereals and breads, gradually increasing the amount of wholegrain foods as your child gets older.

Grains

There are many reasons to eat more whole grains. They:

* contain protein
* are high in complex carbohydrates and fibre
* are low in fat
* contain important antioxidants, vital for health
* provide energy
* protect the body against heart disease
* are economical, easy to cook and highly versatile

Cereals and grains have been a part of our diet for centuries, with different grains being used in different parts of the world. Nowadays, the two most popular grains, worldwide, are wheat (used in bread, pasta and couscous) and rice, but there are many others worth trying. As each grain contains slightly different nutrients, aim to incorporate a range of grains in your family's diet—increasing servings of whole grains as your child gets older —to ensure the best possible nutrition and to help protect your family against cardiovascular disease, diabetes and possibly obesity.

Rice There are several kinds to choose from, depending on recipe requirements. Short grain brown rice is the most nutritious and has a delicious nutty flavour and chewy texture, but there is also long grain brown and white rice, short grain white rice (used in puddings), fragrant basmati rice (the perfect accompaniment to Indian dishes), arborio rice (for creamy risottos), and even red and black rice. Cooking times will vary, so check the packet.

Take care with leftover cooked rice as it can contain bacteria which may cause food poisoning if left at room temperature for any length of time. To avoid this:
* Serve it immediately after cooking.
* Cool any leftovers within an hour and refrigerate until needed.
* Don't keep cooked rice for longer than two days.
* Never re-heat rice more than once.

To cook perfect basmati rice

* After years of cooking rice, I have finally found a way to ensure perfectly cooked, fluffy basmati rice. The basic ration is 3:8, so for 80 g (3 oz) of white rice you need 175 ml (8 fl oz) of boiling water or stock. This can be doubled, tripled or quadrupled, so for 175 g (6 oz) of rice you need 350 ml (16 fl oz) of boiling water, and so on. Fry the rice in a teaspoon of vegetable oil for a minute or so in a saucepan over a medium heat. Add the boiling water or stock (you could use a teaspoon of vegetable bouillon powder), turn the heat right down, put a well-fitting lid on the pan, and simmer very gently for 15 minutes. Turn the heat off and allow the rice to sit for five minutes before using.
* Brown rice takes longer than white rice to cook, and may need to simmer in stock or water for 30 to 40 minutes until it is tender.
* Brown rice contains more vitamins and minerals than white, but the phytic acid in the bran inhibits the absorption of iron and calcium. Easy-cook brown rice has some of the bran removed, making it a better alternative for young children. Soaking brown rice overnight improves its digestibility.

Barley This grain is used in soups, bakes and casseroles to provide a lovely chewy, slightly nutty texture. It can also be used to replace rice in dishes such as risotto. To speed cooking time, soak the barley for eight hours before cooking.

Quinoa Classed as a grain, quinoa is an amazingly nutritious food as it is one of the few non-animal complete proteins, containing all the essential amino acids, as well as being an excellent source of complex carbohydrates. Quinoa has a distinctive light, crisp texture, a slightly nutty flavour and is easy to cook. Simmer one part rinsed quinoa with two parts boiling water or stock for 15–20 minutes in a covered pan, until the water is absorbed and the grain is tender. Use in any dish which calls for couscous or as an alternative to rice.

Millet Like quinoa, this is a small round grain, which can be used in place of couscous or rice. Gluten-free, and a good source of protein, millet has a denser, more floury texture than quinoa, but can be cooked in a similar way. For a nuttier flavour, dry-fry the grain for a minute before adding boiling water or stock. Millet flakes can also be used to thicken soups, added to fruit smoothies, or combined with oats in flapjacks.

Bulghar wheat Also sold as cracked wheat, this is extremely easy to prepare as it just sits in a covered bowl of boiling water or stock for about 20 minutes, until the water has been absorbed. It has a distinctive nutty taste and slightly chewy texture. Use to replace rice or to make salads such as tabbouleh.

Couscous This is not actually a grain but is made from durum wheat, like pasta. However, like grains, it is easy to cook, has a fluffy texture and combines with all sorts of sauces. It is also extremely popular with most children.

Oats Although not used as a whole grain, oats should be used in your cooking wherever possible. An excellent source of dietary fibre, they contain antioxidants, help lower cholesterol, contain anti-inflammatory compounds and provide slow-release carbohydrate. An excellent all-round choice, use rolled oats to make porridge for one of the best energy-giving starts to the day, and in all kinds of baking.

Pasta: what's the alternative?
Try substituting grains such as quinoa, millet, barley and bulghar wheat in your favourite pasta dishes. Barley and millet go well with rich tomato and meat-based sauces. The more delicate flavour of quinoa works well with fish and prawns.

Wheat Bread is one of the most common ways to eat wheat.

* Aim to vary the kinds of bread you buy, choosing wholegrain bread where possible.
* Try making your own bread (see page 226). It is a wonderful activity to share with children and the loaf you produce will be delicious, free from added preservatives and far superior to any shop-bought bread,.
* Rye bread is a dark, dense loaf with a distinctive flavour. Try toasting it and topping with pure fruit spread, or grated cheese and sliced tomatoes.
* Sourdough bread is made without yeast to give a dense, chewy loaf which is excellent toasted.
* Look out for seeded bread, fruit bread, soda bread, scones, wraps, bagels, naans and pittas.
* Serve savoury muffins (see page 216) with soup as an alternative to bread.

Pulses

These are a good source of protein and an essential substitute for meat in vegetarian diets. They also:

* are low in saturated fats
* contain fibre, which may help reduce cholesterol levels in the blood
* count as one portion of the recommended 'five-a-day' fruit and vegetables
* are economical
* provide interesting texture and flavour to familiar recipes

Homemade breadcrumbs

Homemade bread doesn't keep for as long as shop-bought bread, but any leftover slices can be blitzed in a liquidiser or food processor to make breadcrumbs. Store these in the freezer and use to coat fishcakes, strips of fish or chicken, or as a crunchy topping for pasta bakes, fish pies or cauliflower cheese.

Lentils These are a wonderfully convenient food as they are extremely versatile and easy to use. Like all pulses, lentils absorb the flavour of any spices used during cooking, and once boiled until soft they can be served as an accompaniment to meat and fish dishes, or as a component of vegetarian recipes.

There are several different kinds of lentil:

* Red lentils are the quickest to cook. They reduce to a soft mush, making them suitable for soups, pasta sauces and dhal, and also to bulk out and thicken stews and casseroles.
* Brown and green lentils are larger and provide an earthy richness to casseroles. They are also great for salads.
* Puy lentils are small, blue-grey in colour and considered the most sophisticated of lentils. They retain their shape after cooking and have a more delicate flavour. Suitable as an accompaniment to fish, meat and poultry, or as a base for salads.

Soaking pulses

Dried pulses are usually soaked before cooking.
Here's the method I use:

* Soak the dried beans for at least 12 hours – usually overnight.
* Drain and rinse the beans under running water then place in a saucepan and cover them with fresh water.
* Boil the beans vigorously for at least 10 minutes, with the lid off.
* Simmer the beans until tender. Kidney beans take approximately 45–60 minutes; soya beans take two to three hours. You may need to add more water as it boils away.

Pulses which are usually soaked include kidney beans, soya beans, chickpeas, butter beans, cannellini beans, haricot beans, black eye beans and aduki beans.

Adding a teaspoon of bicarbonate of soda to the soaking and cooking water speeds up the process and reduces the cooking time, however it causes a loss of some nutrients. Don't add salt to beans while they are cooking as this toughens the skins.

Not all pulses require soaking, however. Some just need boiling for 20–30 minutes until tender. There is no need to soak lentils (red, brown, green or Puy), mung beans, or green and yellow split peas. However, you can soak split peas for a few hours to speed up the cooking time and reduce the need to skim foam from the surface during cooking.

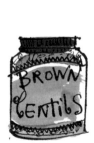
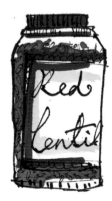
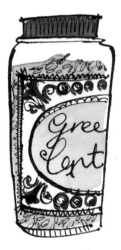
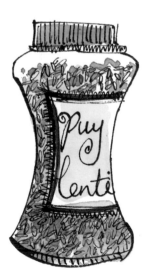

More about pulses

* Once they have been soaked and cooked, pulses will at least double in weight.
* Serve pulses with foods or drinks rich in vitamin C, such as orange juice, berries or peppers, as this aids absorption of the iron present in pulses.
* Cooked pulses should be kept in the fridge and eaten within two days.
* Adding pulses to meat-based dishes makes the finished dish lower in fat and more economical as you will need to use less meat.

Prepare large quantities of pulses and freeze them, once cold, in small portions, ready for immediate use in soups, sauces and casseroles.

Recipes using grains and pulses:

Chickpeas in Tomato Sauce (page 164)
Hearty Bean Soup (page 180)
Carrot, Lentil and Sweet Potato Soup (page 187)
Creamy Vegetarian Lasagne (page 200)
Pot-roast Herby Lamb with Cannellini Beans and Salsa Verde (page 204)
Vegetarian Rice (page 206)
Prawn Risotto (page 211)
Baked Barley Risotto (page 212)
Baked Fish with Quinoa and Roasted Tomatoes (page 213)
Oaty Breakfast Pancakes (page 215)
Fruity Flapjacks (page 217)
Oatcakes (page 222)
Red Pepper Hummus (page 220)
Tomato Bean Dip (page 221)
Roasted Vegetables with Couscous (page 174)
Fish and Prawn Pie with Crunchy Oat Topping (page 197)

Chapter 2
Healthy Eating Made Easy

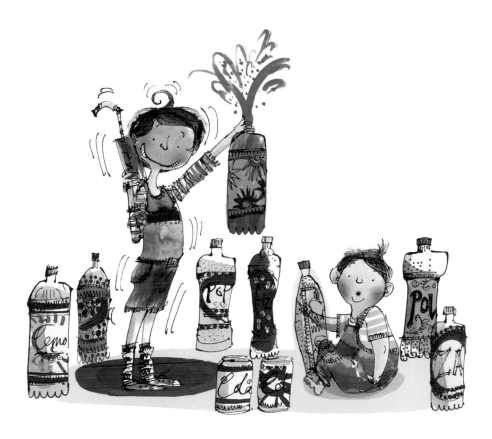

Developing Healthy Eating Habits

Good food and healthy eating habits are essential elements for a happy life, so it is invaluable that you provide your child with these from the very beginning of their introduction to solid food and family meals.

As children are growing and developing faster than they will at any other time of their lives, it is vital that their nutritional requirements are satisfied. These days there is so much conflicting advice about what constitutes a healthy diet and such an abundance of 'ready-meals' claiming to be what you and your family need, that it can be difficult for parents to know what to feed their children.

Basically, the nutrients essential for healthy growth and development are: carbohydrates, proteins, fat, vitamins, minerals and trace elements. These are all found in the four main food groups:

* milk and dairy products, such as yoghurt and cheese
* carbohydrates or starchy foods, such as potatoes, bread, pasta, rice and other grains
* meat and meat alternatives, including, poultry, fish, pulses, eggs, nuts, quinoa and soya
* fruit and vegetables, including root vegetables, leafy green vegetables, salad vegetables, and all fruit and fruit juices

There is a fifth food group of what I consider to be occasional food. This includes cakes, sweet biscuits, crisps, etc. These foods do not form a necessary part of your child's diet as they are generally highly processed and are high in sugar, salt and fat, which can lead to weight problems and high blood pressure later in life. Avoid processed snacks wherever possible and instead develop the habit of offering your child healthy snacks (see page 101). If you wish to offer cakes and biscuits for an occasional tea-time or party treat, have a go at making your own (see Recipes section, pages 163–232). There are many benefits:

* You will know exactly what ingredients are in the treats you make.
* There will be no additives such as colouring, flavouring or artificial sweeteners, which may have an adverse effect on the health and behaviour of susceptible children.
* Your child will develop a preference for less sweet, homemade treats.
* You can enjoy baking with your child and reap the rewards of watching your child's pleasure at cooking together and eating what they have made.
* You can impart an appreciation of homemade food and a love of cooking to your child from an early age.

If you ensure that you offer your child food from all four groups at every meal, you will be giving him a well-balanced diet, containing all the essential nutrients. To achieve optimum nutrition, it is important to provide a range of different foods and not to keep offering the same familiar favourites. To help you achieve this, the recipes in this book make use of a variety of ingredients, as well as suggesting alternatives that can be substituted if you want to try something different.

By preparing nutritious meals and snacks for your child, you will be establishing all-important healthy eating habits from the outset. As well as avoiding highly-processed food and additives, which I find can trigger health, behavioural and sleep problems in some children, you will also be laying firm foundations for enjoyment of good home-cooked, healthy food. Children who are offered a varied diet are less likely to become fussy eaters, but, nevertheless, many children do go through a period of fussiness. This should be short-lived, however, and you can be confident meanwhile that you are providing excellent nutrition and have not caused your child's fussiness by offering ready-made foods and processed snacks, laden with salt, sugar and empty calories. By following the recipes in this book and continuing to offer your child delicious meals and tasty snacks, you should be able to come through the fussy phase without too much frustration (see pages 118–21).

Understanding labels

Eating healthily starts with shopping healthily, and shopping healthily starts with reading and understanding labels. The labels are the equivalent of the small print in a contract; they contain all the information you need to know about the food you're buying. If you want to eat healthily, become an avid reader of the small print, and avoid relying on the health claims on the front of the pack. The better you become at reading labels, the quicker you can sort healthy from unhealthy food.

The most informative label is the list of ingredients. Food that is good for you should contain simple, clear ingredients, much like the ones you would have used had you cooked the dish at home. For the same reason, steer clear of lengthy lists. Nutritious food invariably contains fewer rather than more ingredients.

The list is arranged in descending order, with the ingredient in the largest quantity first and the smallest last. Use that as a quick reference. If the first or second ingredient is sugar or fat, this food item is likely to be unhealthy.

Check how many E numbers the list contains. E numbers, or additives, are required in the commercial production of food to ensure a long shelf life, flavour, look and texture. Their presence in food means that the item was processed, removed from its natural state and made convenient and possibly not healthy. The longer the list of additives, the more processed and therefore less healthy the food. Many food additives have been linked to hyperactivity and behavioural problems in children, as well as allergies and breathing problems. In the interest of health, I believe the consumption of additives should be limited to an absolute minimum. Therefore, look for a short and preferably additive-free list.

If you don't understand what the ingredients on the list are, don't eat them.

Sugar and salt

Sugar and salt are also additives – though not often thought of as such – and are best avoided.

Sugar Look for the 'no added sugar' or 'unsweetened' label, and check the list of ingredients for sugar disguised under another name, such as sucrose, glucose, fructose, maltose, corn syrup and honey. If any of these are high on the list, the product probably has a high sugar content. Up to 10 g (approximately ⅓ oz) sugar (marked as carbohydrates) per 100 g (approximately 3 ½ oz) would be a tolerable amount.

Salt About 75 per cent of the salt we take in comes from processed foods. In other words, most of the salt we eat is already in the foods we buy. This makes it extra-important to check labels whenever possible. Salty-tasting foods, such as salted crisps or ham, are not the only ones high in salt. Foods not thought of as salty, such as some breakfast cereals, can also contain a very high level of salt.

When reading labels, the amount may be given as salt or as sodium, which is one of the chemical components in salt. This can be confusing, but you simply multiply the sodium value by 2.5 to get the salt value. Look at the salt or sodium value per 100 g (3 ½ oz) of the food:

---

* 1.25 g salt or 0.5 g sodium or more means that the food is high in salt.
* 0.25 g salt or 0.1 g sodium or less means that the food is low in salt.

Current government recommendations for salt intake for small children are:
* 1–3 years: a maximum of 2 g salt or 0.8 g sodium per day.
* 4–6 years: a maximum of 3 g salt or 1.2 g sodium per day.

However, be aware that this is a maximum – it is much better for children to have a lower level than this.

Children under two years of age should not have salt added to their food. They get all the salt they need from natural sources such as vegetables. Adding salt to a young baby's food can be very dangerous as it may put a strain on his immature kidneys. Research also shows that children who develop a taste for salt early in life may be more prone to heart disease later. When your baby reaches the stage of joining in with family meals, it is important that you do not add salt to the food during cooking. Remove your baby's portion, then add salt for the rest of the family if necessary. As with sugar, many processed foods and commercially prepared meals contain high levels of salt. It is important to check the labels on these foods carefully before giving them to your toddler.

Remember that unprocessed foods such as fruit, vegetables, grains, pulses, milk, eggs, fish, meat and poultry contain very little or no salt.

Fat

The levels and type of fat are also crucial for health. While children under two need higher levels of fat, above this age you can slowly start to reduce it. For children over five, am to keep general fat levels low, at 3 g or less per 100 g. Saturated fat, whether of animal or plant origin, should also be kept low. Steer clear of any product containing partially or fully hydrogenated fats, which act in a similar way to saturated fat in the body. Inferior quality refined oils are also best avoided. Omega-3, on the other hand, is a healthy and important fatty acid, so it's a good idea to buy products containing it. (See page 64 for more information on omega-3.)

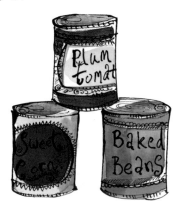

The Pitfalls of Processed Foods

The term 'processed' merely applies to anything that has been done to the food to make it more palatable, digestible or last longer.

Simple techniques, such as heating in sealed jars or cans, salting, milling and drying, have been around for centuries. However, in the current system of food manufacture and retailing, where huge quantities and variety of food are available, and indeed demanded, by the consumer, food processing has become very sophisticated.

*The less sugar and salt your child eats,
the less he will crave it.*

In general, most convenience foods, such as snacks, biscuits, cakes, 'cook-in' sauces, breakfast cereals and 'ready-meals' rely on three main ingredients to increase shelf life and palatability. These are salt, sugar and fats (often hydrogenated). Some of these foods have little or no nutritional value other than calories, and in large amounts they may have adverse affects on health. If eaten frequently children will become accustomed to the taste of these ingredients and an unhealthy pattern is set for life.

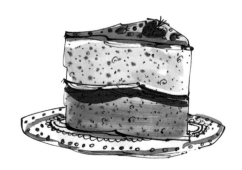

In addition to salt, sugar and fats, many chemical and modified ingredients may be added to these foods to increase shelf life and improve appearance. These can include:

* potassium sorbate	* sulphites
* humectants	* maltodextrin
* sulphur dioxide	* annatto
* emulsifiers	* stabilisers
* tripotassium phosphate	* adipic acid
* acidity regulators	* glucose syrup

Putting aside the claims of adverse health effects or otherwise of these types of ingredients, do you really want to be feeding unrecognisable chemicals to your children? Making your own food, using fresh and simple ingredients, will mean you have control over what your family is eating.

However, some of the more basic processed foods can be nutritious and a boon to a busy mother.

* Simple canned items, such as pulses, fish and tomatoes, are only processed as much as is required to ensure the safety of the product and will retain much of their nutrient value. Try to choose items without added sugar or salt.

* Basic foods such as bread and pasta vary. Choose more wholegrain products as your child gets older to increase nutrient value and keep children feeling full for longer.

* Frozen vegetables are handy and the next best thing to fresh. A handful of peas thrown into a risotto or pasta dish can add colour, flavour and nutrients, for example. Good-quality fish and meat, frozen from fresh, can also be useful.

Suggestions for avoiding processed foods

* For breakfast. Many manufactured cereals contain high levels of salt and sugar. Be sure to read the labels carefully to compare different products or make your own muesli with rolled oats, dried fruit and chopped nuts to a recipe your children enjoy. Try chopped, dried mango, dried cranberries and other exciting ingredients they like. Freshly made porridge with added raisins or banana and perhaps just a little cream or Greek yoghurt is delicious.
* In place of 'breaded' items such as chicken nuggets or fish fingers, dip turkey fillet steaks, chicken breast strips or fish fillet strips into beaten egg and coat in lightly seasoned oatbran or fine oatmeal. Shallow fry or bake.
* Make your own pastry from half wholemeal and half plain flour. Make double quantities and freeze what you do not need.
* Homemade biscuits, muffins and simple cakes are much better snacks for children, using basic ingredients that are wholesome and nutritious.
* Make your own food 'convenient'. Fresh tomato and meat sauces can be made in generous amounts and frozen for another day or converted into another meal. So, mince can make spaghetti Bolognese one day; add kidney beans and a little chilli and you have chilli con carne. A roast chicken one day can become a filling for wraps the next day and added to risotto the day after.

Remember: it is better to provide children with a fresh and varied diet than to rely on highly processed foods with added 'healthy' ingredients.

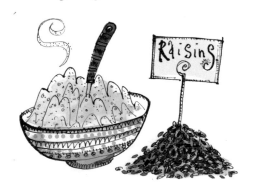

Homemade alternatives

Many processed foods that are sold for children can be easily made at home in healthier and tastier versions. These also have the added advantage that the child can help in the making of their food. For some ideas see the recipes for Lamb Burgers, Favourite Fishcakes, Turkey Burgers and Chicken Pitta Pockets on pages 166, 176, 177 and 178.

Wraps

Children love to design and roll their own wraps, so assemble the ingredients in individual bowls, then let them help themselves and have fun wrapping.

Suggested ingredients

*   cooked chicken torn into strips (hot or cold)
*   shredded lettuce or watercress
*   cucumber and spring onions sliced thinly lengthways
*   fresh tomato salsa or sliced tomatoes
*   sweetcorn kernels
*   sour cream
*   grated mild Cheddar cheese
*   warmed flour tortillas

Other options include cooked mince or Bolognese sauce (reduced so it's not too runny; see recipe for Minced Beef Cobbler, page 194), refried beans and guacamole (see page 221).

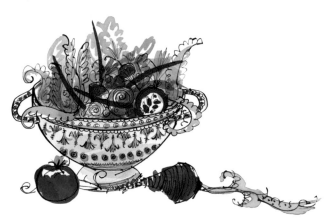

Healthy Drinks

Finding a healthy drink for your child on the supermarket shelves can be difficult. There are rows and rows of enticing bottles in many tempting flavours and bright colours, and children are drawn by these as well as by the familiar brands advertised on television.

The soft drinks industry is a multi-million-pound business, but, unfortunately, most of the drinks produced are quite harmful to children, containing high quantities of sugar which can rot teeth and lead to excessive weight gain. They also often contain artificial additives – colourings and flavourings – which may cause hyperactivity and behavioural problems in some children.

Get into the habit of reading labels, and steer clear of additive-laden drinks.

Artificially sweetened drinks

The alternative to sugary drinks are 'sugar-free' drinks, containing artificial sweeteners, but I would advise caution with these as well. One of the most widely used sweeteners, aspartame, has been linked to all kinds of symptoms such as dizziness, nausea, headaches and hyperactivity. Another one to look out for is cyclamate. While levels of aspartame and cyclamate in bought drinks will be within recommended safe limits, I recommend you avoid artificial sweeteners wherever possible. Encourage your child to develop a taste for the natural sweetness in foods and drinks, such as pure fruit juice.

The Foods Standards Agency advises parents to give young children aged between one and four-and-a-half years old no more than three cups a day (about 180 ml/ 6 fl oz) of dilutable soft drinks containing cyclamate.

Fruit juice

* Fresh fruit juices found in the chiller cabinet are the next best thing to making your own fresh juice.
* The next best option is pure fruit juice made from concentrate. This may not provide quite so many vitamins, as some could be destroyed when the juice is heated to evaporate the water.
* Avoid cartons of drink masquerading as fruit juice. If the carton says 'drink' rather than 'juice', then it will not be pure juice but will probably have added sugar and water and is best left on the shelf.

The fresher the juice, the more nutrients it is likely to contain, so look for the words 'freshly-squeezed' on packaging.

Tips for healthier drinks

* Offer up to one cup (150 ml/5 fl oz) per day of pure fruit juice instead of squash or fizzy drinks. Although all these drinks contain sugar, which can lead to excessive weight gain and contribute to dental caries, pure fruit juice also contains useful nutrients, such as vitamin C.
* Make your child smoothies by blending fruit on its own, or adding a little milk.
* If your child has to have fruit juice, it is best to offer it at mealtimes. A small amount of fruit juice with meals also helps the iron in food to be absorbed because of the vitamin C the juice contains.
* Drinks other than water given in baby bottles cause increased dental decay, as the juice is in prolonged contact with the teeth. Try to wean your baby off the bottle by introducing a cup at six months. Do not allow your child to go to bed with a bottle, as this is associated with high levels of dental caries and there is also a risk of choking.
* If you limit your child to 150 ml (5 fl oz) of pure fruit juice per day, it will keep his sugar intake to a reasonable level and count (only once a day) as one portion of the recommended five daily portions of fruit and vegetables.
* Offer water or milk rather than sugary drinks. If children insist on fruit juice, dilute it with water (in a ratio of 1:5) to make it less sugary (and last longer).

* Get your child to brush his teeth after a sugary drink.
* Children like drinking out of trendy sports-type bottles, so try filling them with water.

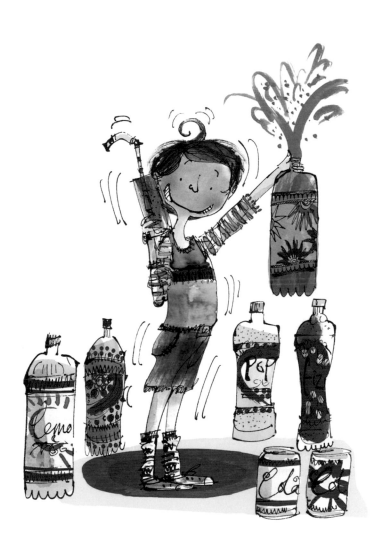

Omega-3 and Omega-6 Essential Fatty Acids

Omega-3 fats: brain food

Omega-3 fats, like vitamins and minerals, are essential for your child's development. These are the healthy fats that are contained in oil-rich fish such as salmon and sardines. Many people associate omega-3s with a decreased risk of heart disease in adults, but they have many other roles besides and are a critical component of nerve tissues. During a child's time in the womb and through the rapid growth of the first years of life, his body uses these essential fats to build a healthy brain, eyes and other nerve tissues such as the adrenal glands (responsible for making certain hormones) and testicular tissue. It is estimated that 70 per cent of the brain's growth occurs while a baby is in the womb, the next 15 per cent during infancy, and the remaining 15 per cent during the pre-school years. As you can imagine, having enough omega-3 fat is therefore of great importance throughout this period of rapid development. It is reflected in the fact that a good intake of omega-3s by mothers during pregnancy seems to help babies develop well in areas such as growth, visual ability and mental processing (and may also help to prevent postnatal depression in the mother). Similar benefits have been seen in children who are breastfed (breast milk is rich in omega-3s, particularly if the mother has a good omega-3 intake herself) or given infant formulas containing omega-3s. It seems the old saying that fish is brain food is true.

The effect of omega-3 fats doesn't stop there. They are involved in the production of hormone-like substances that regulate a whole host of body functions. Registered dietitian Fiona Hinton reports: 'As far as children are concerned, there's research into a wide range of possible benefits from omega-3 fats, including reductions in allergy risk and improvements in behavioural problems and developmental disorders. There's even speculation among some scientists that there may be a link between low omega-3 intake and persistent bedwetting!'

Areas which scientists are currently investigating include:
* attention deficit (hyperactivity) disorder (ADHD)
* dyslexia
* developmental coordination disorder (DCD), also known as dyspraxia
* autistic spectrum disorders
* childhood depression
* immune function
* asthma
* allergies
* type 1 (childhood) diabetes
* persistent bedwetting

Scientists have even said that a good intake of omega-3 fats in the pre-school years may enhance children's ability to learn. While research into these areas is still in the early stages, it's important that all children receive adequate omega-3 fats to be sure of optimal brain and nervous system development and to reap any potential benefits.

What are omega-3s and where do we find them?

Omega-3s are a specific type of fat. All types of fat are similar, but small differences in the structure of their molecules bring very different health effects. The omega-3 fats are a member of the family known as 'polyunsaturated'. The other member is omega-6. Together these fats comprise the 'essential' fats, which means that we must take these fats in through our diet in order for our bodies to function properly.

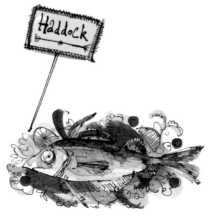

By far the best food source of omega-3 fats is fish, but only the types known as 'oily' or 'oil-rich' fish. The most common are:

* salmon
* trout
* mackerel
* herring
* sardines
* pilchards
* kipper
* eel
* whitebait
* tuna (fresh only)
* anchovies
* swordfish
* bloater
* carp
* orange roughy
* sprats

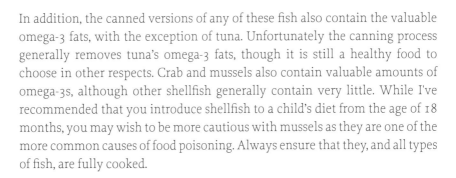

In addition, the canned versions of any of these fish also contain the valuable omega-3 fats, with the exception of tuna. Unfortunately the canning process generally removes tuna's omega-3 fats, though it is still a healthy food to choose in other respects. Crab and mussels also contain valuable amounts of omega-3s, although other shellfish generally contain very little. While I've recommended that you introduce shellfish to a child's diet from the age of 18 months, you may wish to be more cautious with mussels as they are one of the more common causes of food poisoning. Always ensure that they, and all types of fish, are fully cooked.

I suggest that you don't offer smoked fish more than once a week as it is high in salt and a chemical called nitrate. Nitrate can change to potentially harmful substances in our digestive system, but having a source of vitamin C at the same meal, such as fresh tomato or a satsuma, prevents this conversion.

Non-fish sources of omega-3

While oil-rich fish are the best source of omega-3s, there are other foods that supply them.

* In larger supermarkets you will find eggs that contain omega-3 fats, which are produced by feeding the chickens a special diet. Do note that regular eggs are not a good source of omega-3s. Eggs with omega-3 will be clearly labelled, and may mention being heart-healthy.
* Flaxseeds and flaxseed oil (also known as linseeds and linseed oil): the oil, while quite high in plant omega-3s, has a strong taste and is not suitable for cooking. Children may not notice it when drizzled over other quite strong-tasting foods such as homemade pizza or spaghetti Bolognese. The seeds can be ground and sprinkled on cold or hot cereals, or you can look for 'split' seeds and mix them into yoghurt or fruit juice. Start with small amounts, as they are high in fibre and may upset younger digestive systems.
* Walnuts and walnut oil: the oil is not suitable for cooking but is delicious used on salads. Children may prefer the nut itself (assuming they are old enough and there is no risk of allergy), possibly sprinkled on cereal, salads or desserts, or added to muffins and cakes. Be sure to chop nuts finely for younger children.
* Rapeseed oil is a good choice for general cooking. It's often found in the supermarket simply labelled as 'vegetable oil' so you may need to check the ingredient list.
* Soy-based foods such as tofu.
* Spirulina, a type of seaweed.

The advantage of omega-3 eggs over the other, plant-based omega-3 sources is that the eggs contain the types of omega-3 found in fish, particularly DHA. This is the type used to build brains and thought to be responsible for many of the health benefits. While our bodies can convert the type found in plant foods to the types found in fish, in practice we convert very little. This means you need a very large amount of plant-type omega-3 to supply useful amounts of fish-type omega-3s.

Omega-3 fats are being added to a small but increasing range of commonly consumed foods such as milk and probiotic drinks. These will be particularly useful for children who can't, or don't want to, eat fish. Note that some probiotic drinks state that they should be used only by children over the age of three.

Top tip

Store walnuts, walnut oil, flaxseeds and flaxseed oil in the fridge to prevent the oils becoming rancid or going 'off'.

More omega-3 for all the family

The recommendation from the British Food Standards Agency is to eat at least one portion of oil-rich fish each week. An adult portion of fish is 140 g (about 4.5 oz) but children will eat a smaller portion size; this will range from just a few teaspoons of fish up to an adult-sized serving, depending on age and appetite. According to dietitian Fiona Hinton, few adults or children meet this recommendation: 'It really worries me that most people eat very little oil-rich fish, on average only about a third of a portion each week, meaning that both we and our children may be missing out on the benefits of omega-3 fats.' People often avoid cooking fish because they think it may be difficult, but it is actually the basis for really quick, easy meals. And with the convenience of canned salmon or sardines, there's really no reason not to include oil-rich fish in your family's diet once or twice each week.

Some children don't like the taste of fish. If that's the case, try to disguise it with other flavours. For example, gently stir fry chunks of salmon with vegetables, noodles, a drizzle of honey, and a squeeze of lemon juice or splash of low-salt soy sauce.

You can also tempt younger children by making fun fishy foods:

* Mix cooked mackerel with cream cheese and a little lemon juice. Spread it on a flatbread and top with grated carrot and grated cheese. Roll up the flatbread, then slice it into pinwheels.
* Make a face on a round piece of bread using chopped vegetables, meats and cheese. Add pink salmon lips and a nose made of mackerel or fresh tuna.

Precautions

Fish can be contaminated with mercury, a dangerous type of metal, as well as other substances. These can be particularly dangerous to the development of babies and young children. Therefore, it is recommended that girls and women up to and during childbearing age limit oil-rich fish to no more than two portions per week, while boys, men, and women beyond childbearing age may eat up to four portions per week. In addition, children under the age of 16 should not be offered shark, swordfish or marlin because these fish contain higher levels of mercury that could affect development of the nervous system. Fish is a very healthy food, but you can get too much of a good thing.

Omega-3 supplements

There are a number of omega-3 supplements available and this can seem a good option for those who can't or don't eat much fish. However, dietitians recommend that children receive their omega-3s from fish if possible as we don't eat fish just for the omega-3s. Fish is a very nutritious, protein-rich food that also supplies valuable vitamins and is our best source of the mineral iodine.

If you do feel that a supplement is required, speak to your GP regarding the amount and type of omega-3s it supplies. As with oil-rich fish, too much of these supplements can be harmful. Most omega-3 supplements are made from fish oils and may not be suitable for those with allergies or for vegetarians. There is a supplement available that contains the valuable DHA form of omega-3 which is made from algae, and which will be acceptable to strict vegetarians.

Omega-6: another essential fat

Omega-6 fats are also essential for our body to function properly. However, unlike omega-3s they are found in many of the foods children eat every day so you don't need to look for more of them or think about supplements. In fact, researchers think that we are eating too much of this type of fat, and that the balance should be shifted to less of these and more omega-3s. The main sources of omega-6 fats are most vegetable oils, including sunflower, safflower and corn oil, margarines and the many processed foods made using these vegetable oils, from ready-made sandwiches to biscuits and crackers. Many seeds and nuts such as pine nuts and sunflower seeds are also rich sources of omega-6 fats.

Omega-3 – the one to choose

Where possible, try to choose oils and other foods rich in omega-3 fats rather than just omega-6. For example, choose rapeseed oil rather than sunflower oil when cooking.

Easy fish meals

Fish can be anything from gourmet restaurant fare to a five-minute supper. Here are five quick and child-friendly ideas to help you put fish on your family's table. Note that the last three ideas can be puréed for babies (although you'll need to leave out the honey), and do remember to remove all bones in children's portions:

* Make salmon sandwiches with cucumber and a squeeze of lemon; younger ones may prefer the salmon mashed with cream cheese.
* Serve sardines on toast topped with warmed chopped tomatoes.
* Grill mackerel fillets then drizzle them with a mixture of honey and fresh orange juice. (Remember that honey is unsuitable for children under one.)
* Mix pasta or rice with canned salmon, frozen cooked vegetables and white sauce.
* Top salmon steaks or fillets with cream cheese mashed with mustard and lemon juice, or with honey. Bake them in a moderate oven until cooked through.

Always discuss any nutritional supplements with a GP before giving them to your child.

Try to make one night a week 'Fish Night'. Then add an easy lunch of a sardine or salmon sandwich on another day and you'll dramatically increase your child's (and the rest of the family's) omega-3 intake.

Recipes containing oily fish:

Mild Salmon and Coconut Curry (page 190)
Salad Niçoise (page 208)
Pasta with Salmon and Broccoli (page 214)
Favourite Fishcakes (page 176)

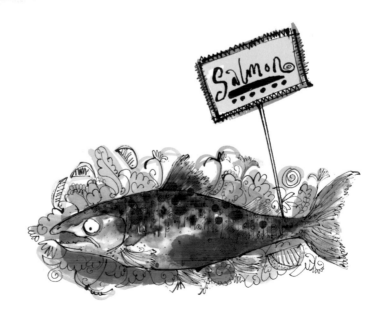

Antioxidants

Antioxidants are natural chemicals found in a variety of foods. It is thought they may protect you and your children in the long term against heart disease, certain cancers and the ageing process.

In the shorter term these nutrients help to protect us from the effects of pollution, toxic exposure to chemicals and sun damage. Key antioxidants include: vitamin C, vitamin E, beta-carotene, anthocyanidins, lutein, lycopene and selenium.

Antioxidants play the housekeeper's role, 'mopping up' free radicals before they get a chance to do harm in your body. Free radicals are unstable, reactive particles naturally created in our bodies in response to exposure to toxins, cigarette smoke and sun damage. Once formed, free radicals can start a chain reaction, similar to dominoes. They can start to damage cell membranes or even our DNA (the genetic blueprint in all of our cells). It is thought that free-radical damage may lead to problems such as pre-cancerous changes in the long term. Antioxidants destroy these dangerous free radicals.

Vitamin C plays a primary role in the formation of collagen, which is important for the growth and repair of body tissue cells, gums, blood vessels, bones and teeth. It can help children absorb iron, a lack of which can lead to fatigue and poor concentration. Vitamin C-rich foods are also a great idea for children fighting infections. Children love squeezing their own orange juice, which is packed with vitamin C.

A combination of vitamin C and vitamin E may help children who have an inherited tendency towards high cholesterol levels and heart disease. Vitamin E has also been shown to play a role in immune function, and its antioxidant properties help protect the membrane or outer wall of our cells.

Carotenoids are red, orange and yellow pigments in plants and animals. In addition to providing colour, they act as antioxidants, and your body also converts certain ones (beta-carotene is the most common) into vitamin A, which is essential for eye health and good immune function. It promotes growth, strong bones and healthy skin. See page 187 for a delicious carotenoid-rich carrot, lentil and sweet potato soup.

Blueberries and red grapes are good sources of anthocyanidins. They improve cellular antioxidant defences and may help prevent cancer. They are also excellent at reducing inflammation. A mixed berry fruit salad is a great idea for picnics or packed lunches.

Lycopene is a carotenoid that provides the red colour to tomatoes, guavas, rosehips, watermelon and pink grapefruit. It is a great antioxidant to prevent cell damage and may protect against prostate cancer. Research shows that lycopene in tomatoes can be absorbed more efficiently by the body if they are processed into juice, sauce, paste and ketchup. The chemical form of lycopene found in tomatoes is converted by the temperature changes involved in processing to make it more easily absorbed by the body. So canned tomatoes actually contain more lycopene than fresh ones – and make a great pasta sauce.

Lutein is the pigment found in dark green leafy vegetables such as spinach and broccoli. Egg yolks are also sources of lutein. It provides nutritional support to your children's eyes and scientists have suggested that it may protect against the development of cataracts. If your child has poor eyesight you may want to focus on giving them lutein-rich foods. A broccoli quiche is easy and popular with children.

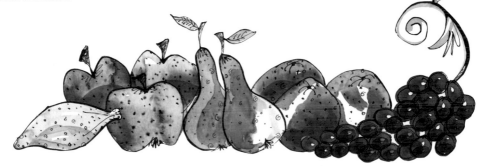

Selenium is a mineral known to have antioxidant properties and seems to work in concert with vitamin E in this respect. It is also involved in healthy immune system activity and may play a role in recovery from viruses. If your child has a virus you might want to offer a couple of brazil nuts as a snack, as they are by far the richest source of selenium.

Antioxidant-rich foods:

Vitamin C
Look for red, orange and green peppers, broccoli, cantaloupe melons, kiwis, oranges, satsumas, clementines, strawberries, tomatoes.

Vitamin E
Almonds, avocadoes, peanut butter, walnuts, wheat germ, vegetable oils (e.g. sunflower oil) and margarines made from them, spinach, kale, broccoli.

Beta-carotene
Look for orange sweet potatoes, cantaloupe melons, carrots, butternut squash, pumpkin, mangoes, spinach, kale, broccoli.

Anthocyanidins
Look for red, blue and purple berries, cherries, red grapes.

Lycopene
Look for red and orange tomatoes (including tomato juice, tomato sauce and tinned tomatoes), watermelons, guavas, papayas, apricots, pink grapefruits.

Lutein
Look for bright green spinach, kale, broccoli, chard.

Selenium
Look for brazil nuts, fish and shellfish, liver, beef, pork, chicken, brown rice, wholewheat bread.

Boosting the Immune System

Every minute of the day children are exposed to germs in their environment. Right from birth a child's body adopts strategies to deal with them, collectively called the immune system.

This amazing piece of engineering is a complex maze of interconnecting organs and cells including the lymphatic system, spleen and bone marrow. The immune system is often described as an army, as there are so many forces working together to protect our bodies from disease by attacking unwanted intruders such as viruses, bacteria, fungi and cancer cells. A lack of certain vitamins and minerals, or too many of the wrong kind of nutrients, may cause the immune system to function much less effectively.

Signs of a lowered immune system

Signs of a lowered immune system can include: frequent colds and infection, slow wound healing, exhaustion after light exercise, dry skin and eczema, asthma, loss of appetite, white marks on nails, poor growth, pale skin, nausea, fatigue, mouth ulcers, plantar warts, molluscum, pimples on back of arms, poor sleep patterns and slow recovery from colds and infections.

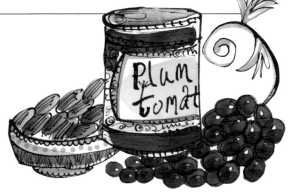

Maintaining a healthy body and immune system

Keep the following points in mind to help strengthen your child's immune system:

1. Increase fruits and vegetables We are all aware that at least five portions of fruit and vegetables are key to maintaining a healthy immune system. Even if your child has decided they don't like fruit and vegetables it is amazing how you can disguise them. Soup, pasta sauces packed with vegetables, or gratingcarrot and courgette into omelettes or muffins are all good strategies for hiding vegetables and making some of the foods they love healthier. Although fresh is best you can also use dried fruit, frozen berries and vegetables, tinned fruit, and baby purées to achieve the five-a-day goal.

2. Limit sugar Some nutritionists have suggested that eating a lot of sugar may impact on a child's immune system. While other health practitioners might debate this, there is no harm and a lot of good ini limiting children's sugar intake.

Remember that sugar is hidden in all sorts of foods under various pseudonyms, mainly ending in 'ose'. They include glucose, glucose syrup, maltose, dextrose, inverted sugar syrup, lactose, golden syrup, honey, corn syrup, treacle, hydrolysed starch, fructose and concentrated fruit juice. Many commercial breakfast cereals are very high in sugar.

3. Drink plenty of water Water is incredibly important for children, both when they are well and when they are under the weather. Proper hydration is one of the fundamentals of health and children who are frequently dehydrated are at increased risk of suffering from headaches and urinary tract infections. When you are off to the park or on a shopping trip always take a bottle of water for each child. Concentration levels are better maintained when water is drunk throughout the day, rather than just at mealtimes. This is why schools often ask parents to provide a water bottle for their child. I believe that filtered water is the best option for your family.

4. Consider probiotics and prebiotics Live yoghurt and probiotic drinks are increasingly popular today. They contain live bacterial cultures, or good bacteria, which many people think is fundamental to our immune systems.

Probiotics means 'for-life'. The digestive tract is home to over four hundred species of micro-organisms. Some are 'good bugs' and some are 'bad bugs' or unhealthy bacteria. Probiotic bacteria are the 'good bugs'. Two of the most common strains are *lactobacilli* and *bifido* bacteria. It is believed that if a positive balance of good bacteria is maintained, the bad bacteria are less able to cause disease and irritation.

Prebiotics are substances that feed probiotics and help them grow and multiply. The main prebiotics are called *inulin* and *oligofructose*, which are found in fibrous foods such as bananas and chicory.

Trials are still in early stages but initial findings hint that adding prebiotic and probiotic food sources to your child's diet may:
* reduce the risk or duration of some types of diarrhoea
* help manage lactose intolerance
* reduce the risk of colon cancer
* reduce prevalence of allergies
* boost the immune response

Sources of prebiotics
Jerusalem artichokes, wheat, barley, rye, onions, leeks, chicory, honey, bananas, cereals with added inulin, some probiotic drinks

Sources of probiotics
Live yoghurt, buttermilk, miso (paste made from fermented rice, barley, or soya beans), kefir (drink made from fermented milk), probiotic drinks

---

Note that many of the probiotic drinks on the market also contain large amounts of sugar or sweeteners and flavourings, so compare brands to make the best choice. Also, some brands recommend against giving the drinks to very youg children, so again, check the label to be sure.

5. *Let them get dirty!* It is thought that children need to be exposed to a certain amount of germs in order to train their immune system to focus its attention on harmful invaders such as bacteria and viruses.

Some scientists who have investigated the anti-bacterial-resistant, so-called 'super bugs', such as MRSA, have suggested that one of the reasons that these microbes have become so widespread in recent years is down to the modern Western obsession with hygiene and the overuse of anti-bacterial products. Obviously the solution isn't to refuse to clean our houses or wash our bodies, but it is worth remembering that soap and water, or natural cleaning products – for example, vinegar and essential oils such as lemon and tea tree – can be perfectly adequate.

Developing Appetite

Many parents are concerned that their children have very small appetites or are unwilling to eat much at all. If you have a reluctant eater on your hands then there are a number of factors which may contribute to this.

Before getting too concerned, it is important to check the following:

* Are your eyes bigger than their tummies? Too much food on a plate can be overwhelming to many children. A rough guide is to look at the size of their palms. One portion equals one palmful. Aim to have one palmful of protein, one palmful of carbohydrate and one palmful of vegetables per meal.
* Are they snacking too much between meals? Snacks can be helpful at supporting energy levels between meals. (Oatcakes for toddler age and above are a great help.) A snack should, however, be a snack, not a mini-meal. One oatcake, or half an apple, or a handful of grapes are a good gauge for most toddlers. Fruit juice between meals can easily curb appetites at mealtimes. Stick to water as much as possible.
* Are they taking enough exercise? Exercise is incredibly important for fuelling the appetite. If your child is a poor eater at lunch, take him to the park or let him run around in your garden for an hour beforehand so that he works up an appetite. If he can go shopping with you by bicycle or tricycle, even better.
* Look for any medical/nutritional indications and raise these with your GP or health visitor.
* A child with uncontrolled reflux or colic may well find eating uncomfortable and associate eating with pain. A parent of a child with reflux or colic needs to work extra hard to build up the child's positive relationship with food.
* Does your child have food allergies/sensitivities? (See page 81 for more on food allergy and intolerance.) Always seek advice on establishing the

food culprits from your GP, paediatrician or dietitian.

* Listen to your child. If he often says he feels sick after eating food, he may well be right. Constipation and/or diarrhoea are also good indicators that the digestive tract is not functioning well. Children who sleep curled up in a ball or on their fronts may be sub-consciously trying to tell you they have a sore stomach.

* Mouth ulcers might be the problem. Even the smallest of mouth ulcers can put anyone off their food. Check your child's mouth, just in case.

* Ensure your child is eating sources of zinc. Zinc helps taste buds to function, as well as boosting the immune system. It is hard to enjoy food if you can't taste or smell it properly.

* Teething can put even the best of eaters off their food. Also check your child has enough teeth to break down the foods you are giving them. We are often in a rush to get them onto 'grown-up' food too quickly.

* Is your child under the weather or going down with a bug? Many of us lose our appetite when ill, and a child is no exception. Don't force a child to eat if he is ill. If you have a child who is recuperating, be gentle and encourage him slowly but surely to eat (see 'Feeding During Illness', page 92) and most importantly, ensure that he is taking in lots of fluids.

* Are they are overtired? This is often why children go off their food or are reluctant eaters. Look for underlying reasons for tiredness such as late bedtimes, or too many play-dates or after-school activities.

Foods to boost zinc levels

Beef, lamb, yoghurt, pork, spinach, chicken, wholegrain bread, turkey, oats, salmon, peas, lentils, milk, brown rice

---

Food Allergy
and Intolerance

What is a food allergy?

A food allergy is an adverse reaction to a specific substance – such as peanuts or fish – that the body perceives as foreign. In their most serious form, food allergies are life-threatening, but at their most subtle they may cause no more than an itchy rash. Whatever form the food allergy takes, finding the cause – or causes – can be very difficult because the average diet includes such a wide range of foods, many of them processed and containing numerous ingredients. Even when the offending substance is known, it can still be difficult to avoid it, especially at social gatherings, in restaurants or on holiday.

Who gets food allergies?

Children under three years of age are more likely than others to develop food allergies, which are diagnosed in 3–7 per cent of children before their third birthday. But the good news is that many outgrow their allergy. By five years of age, 98 per cent of children will lose their allergy to eggs and milk. However, allergies to peanuts and tree nuts (such as almonds, brazil nuts and hazelnuts) are more likely to persist. If your child comes from an allergic (also know as 'atopic') family – if you or your partner, or any of your other children has any kind of allergy, such as hayfever or eczema – he is more likely to develop a food allergy.

Symptoms of food allergies

There are two types of food allergies: immediate (symptoms appear quickly) and delayed (symptoms appear slowly). Food allergies that provoke an immediate reaction (within two hours) are more life-threatening than those producing a delayed reaction, but fortunately are easier to diagnose. Eliminating problem foods is also more straightforward.

Severe allergic reactions

The medical term for a severe allergic reaction is anaphylaxis. Symptoms include:

* swelling of the lips, tongue, mouth or throat
* difficulty swallowing or speaking
* collapse and unconsciousness

If you notice any of these symptoms in your child during or immediately after eating, stop feeding him, call 999 for an ambulance or take him straight to the nearest accident and emergency department. If the symptoms do not seem severe, and you are unsure what to do, call NHS Direct for advice on 0845 4647. It is important to identify the offending food so that it can be avoided in the future. Anaphylactic reactions can be treated whatever the cause, provided you get help quickly.

Delayed reactions

Delayed allergic reactions can cause a wide spectrum of symptoms that may appear up to three days later. Symptoms include:

* reflux
* stomach pain or bloating
* poor growth
* diarrhoea or constipation
* runny or blocked nose
* eczema and asthma

The causes of such allergies are harder to diagnose because of the delayed appearance of symptoms. It is also important to remember that not all the symptoms of delayed reactions are necessarily related to food. Asthma and eczema, for example, might be triggered by pollen or house-dust mites.

Most common food allergies in the UK

Known medically as 'allergens', the most common foods to cause allergies are:

* milk
* wheat
* fish and shellfish
* egg

* soya
* peanuts
* tree nuts (such as almonds, cashews, walnuts, hazelnuts, etc)

If you think your child may have a food allergy of any kind, it is vital that you consult your GP or paediatrician. Managing a child with a true food allergy requires constant vigilance, and helping a young child to understand why he can't have a certain food can be very tricky. However, although food allergy is on the increase, it is important to remember that true food allergy is still quite rare.

What is food intolerance?

Food intolerance has a new medical name: non-allergic food hypersensitivity. This includes a variety of adverse reactions to many different foods or ingredients. Symptoms seem to be worse if larger quantities are consumed. There is often a time delay – up to 72 hours – so it is often difficult to figure out what foods are triggering symptoms.

The reaction is not the same as a food allergy, because it doesn't involve the immune system. It should not be confused with food poisoning either, which is caused by toxic substances that would cause symptoms in anyone who ate the food.

Causes of food intolerance

Food intolerance occurs when the body is unable to deal with a certain type of food. This sometimes happens because the body doesn't produce enough of the particular chemical or enzyme that is needed for digestion of that particular foodstuff. Problems may also occur if a component of food that is not fully digested gets into the blood stream. There are also a number of substances naturally found in our diet that can trigger symptoms. An example is vasoamines, which are found in foods including cheese and chocolate. In addition, some foods, such as shellfish and strawberries can trigger symptoms similar to a true food allergy.

One common culprit is cows' milk, which contains a type of sugar called lactose. Sometimes people have a shortage of the enzyme lactase, which is normally made by cells lining the small intestine. Without this enzyme they can't break down milk sugar into simpler forms that can be absorbed into the bloodstream. Lactose intolerance can cause symptoms very similar to irritable bowel syndrome in adults and colic in babies.

Symptoms of food intolerance

Numerous symptoms of food intolerance have been reported, ranging from migraine and eczema to concentration issues. Symptoms are varied and can include some of the ones in the list below. However, be aware that some of these symptoms can be caused by other things and if you have any concerns you should consult your GP or paediatrician.

* deep-sunk eyes or dark areas around the eyes
* rashes around the mouth or burning in the mouth
* abdominal pain – often shown in a young child or baby who sleeps on their tummy or curled up in a ball
* irregular bowel movements or foul-smelling stools
* linear creases under the eyelids or 'crow's feet'
* bright red ears
* bright red cheeks
* constant rubbing of nose or facial grimacing because the nose, eyes and ears are so itchy
* a fixation on a certain food may also indicate a sensitivity to it

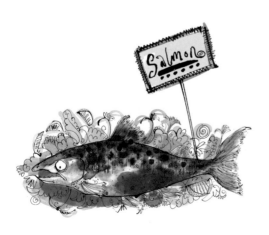

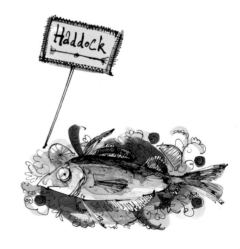

Currently, although research is being carried out in this area, there are no tests available to identify food intolerance correctly: many give false positives, which could encourage a parent to place a child on an unnecessarily restrictive diet. If you think your child might be intolerant of a food, it's best to avoid the food for a few weeks, then reintroduce it and see if the symptoms reappear.

However, if your child has a handful of the above signs and you are concerned about his development, or you are considering eliminating any foods from his diet, he might benefit from pursuing formal evaluation through a GP, paediatrician or dietitian.

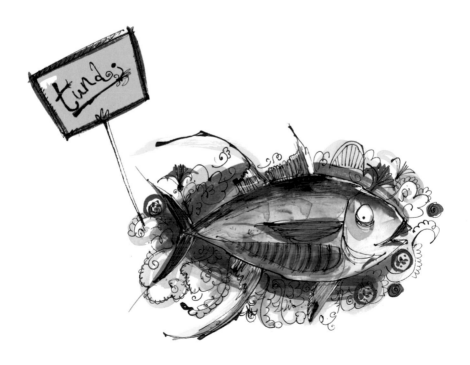

Vegetarian Children

The number of vegetarians in the UK is estimated at 3 million. Food scares and consumers' worries over the safety of their food have helped to push this number up.

A vegetarian is defined as someone living on a plant-based diet, which includes vegetables, fruit, grains, pulses, nuts and seeds, and may also include dairy products and eggs. Strictly speaking, vegetarians do not eat any meat, fowl, game, fish or seafood. Young children, even babies, may show natural aversion to meat or animal flesh. Gradually, as children find out about the connection between their favourite farm animal and the piece of steak on their plate, this aversion may intensify. At teenage (and pre-teenage), insisting on a vegetarian diet can become even more fashionable, as animal-rights issues come to the fore. What seems natural to a child, however, is not always viewed favourably by the parents, who may have strong reservations about the validity of a vegetarian diet.

Children of vegetarian parents may grow up naturally as vegetarians. Both they and their parents feel comfortable with the diet. The issue is more with non-vegetarian parents whose children 'rebel' by refusing the daily meat dish. If you are the parent of such a child, you may feel baffled ('why wouldn't my child eat what the whole family loves?'), concerned (about potential nutrient deficiencies), confused (about the kind of food to offer), and even frustrated (about the need to shop and cook separately for your child). You may doubt the soundness of a vegetarian diet. Even if you as a parent decide to convert the family to vegetarianism, you may still experience some of these feelings, which are perfectly natural for a caring parent.

Many studies have shown that a good vegetarian diet may significantly reduce the risk of heart disease, certain cancers, high blood pressure and obesity. It may also cut down substantially the risk of food poisoning.

It is important to bear in mind that a vegetarian diet can be a perfectly healthy diet throughout life. Practised properly, a plant-based diet provides all the essential protein, minerals, vitamins, fats, fibre and other nutrients essential for good health. In fact, a good vegetarian diet reflects most of the dietary recommendations for healthy eating, being high in fibre, fresh fruit and vegetables and complex carbohydrates, and being low in saturated fat.

The key to a successful vegetarian diet lies in ensuring a good nutrient balance. This is achieved by providing your child with a variety of foods. Use this diagram as a roughguide:

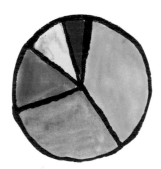

- Vegetables and fruit (40 percent)
- Wholemeal cereals (30 percent)
- Beans, lentils, peas (pulses), Soy products, nuts, Seeds, and eggs (15 percent)
- Dairy products (10 percent)
- Healthy fat (5 percent)

Though these foods ensure a healthy and balanced diet, many parents remain concerned about potential nutrient deficiencies in the vegetarian diet, such as inadequate amounts of protein, vitamin B12, iron or calcium.

Protein appears to be of particular concern. In a vegetarian diet pulses, nuts, seeds, eggs, soy and dairy products are the main protein sources. Grain foods contain some protein, too. These sources provide good easily digestible protein in sufficient quantities for good health. If no animal products are eaten ,a combination of pulses or nuts with grain foods provides protein of the same quality. Soy foods and quinoa are the only plant foods that supply 'complete protein' on their own.

The average Western diet tends to include too much protein in the form of animal flesh that can be high in saturated fat. Replacing some of it with plant protein is beneficial for the family as a whole, and is in line with nutritional recommendations by the UK Heart Association.

Vitamin B12 is an essential vitamin, which the body cannot synthesise by itself. As well as being present in meat, it is in fact available in sufficient quantities from eggs, dairy products and B12-fortified foods. It can also be taken as a supplement following consultation with your GP.

Iron is an important mineral essential for health and energy. Iron deficiency is the most common nutritional deficiency worldwide, regardless of whether people are vegetarian or not. In the vegetarian diet iron is obtainable from green leafy vegetables, pulses, eggs, wholemeal cereals and dried fruit. Iron, from eggs and plant sources, is better absorbed in the presence of vitamin C, so do ensure that you serve vitamin-C-rich foods, such as a glass of orange juice or a tomato salad, alongside iron-rich ones. Studies show that vegetarians are not more iron deficient than meat eaters, though iron stores may be lower.

Calcium is important for bone health. It is found in dairy foods, calcium-fortified soy products, white bread, tofu, pulses, green leafy vegetables, nuts and sesame seeds.

> ### An example of a day's vegetarian menu for a four-year-old:
>
> Breakfast: a fruit, nut and yoghurt smoothie or oat porridge with sliced banana
>
> Snack: a piece of fruit or a handful of dried fruit; or a rice cake with almond butter
>
> Lunch: an egg, lettuce and cress seed-rich sandwich with cherry tomatoes and avocado
>
> Afternoon Snack: a small pot of plain bio-yoghurt with fresh cut fruit
>
> Dinner: lentil soup; baked barley risotto with a green vegetable or a side salad

A good vegetarian diet includes many foods that children, especially young ones, may be unfamiliar with or even resistant to. It is, however, essential that the diet is as inclusive and wholesome as possible to ensure your child receives all the nutrients he needs. A vegetarian diet is not a licence to eat unlimited amounts of cheesy pasta or breakfast cereals with milk.

Making life easier
If you are embarking on life with a vegetarian child there are many ways to ensure a smooth transition to a new way of cooking and eating.

* Invest in a good vegetarian cook book, preferably with a focus on children.
* If your child is old enough, discuss the need to include a variety of different foods if meat is refused.
* Substitute favourite meat dishes with a vegetarian equivalent, for instance: Bolognese sauce made with vegetarian mince; vegetarian instead of meat sausages and burgers; lasagne made with tomatoes, aubergines and mozzarella.
* When you are ready to move on from meat substitutes, explore authentic vegetarian recipes using new ingredients.
* Read and learn about vegetarian eating so you can make informed choices.
* Make gradual changes and go at a pace that you feel comfortable with;

reserve experimentation with new food for the weekend, when you have more time on your hands.

* Decide how far you can and wish to go as a parent. A young child may be indifferent to animal foods if they are not recognisable as such (e.g. meat stock, gelatine, gravy). This allows for more flexibility. An older child or teenager may object to any animal ingredients in his food.
* Switch the whole family onto a vegetarian menu twice a week to reduce the work load.
* Spend more time at the fruit and vegetables section of the supermarket, and ensure these foods account for the bulk of your shopping trolley.
* Visit your local health food store for a variety of fresh and dried produce that may not be available at your supermarket.
* Make occasional use of ready-made vegetarian meals and sauces to ease the transition.
* Attend cooking workshops to learn about new foods and cooking methods.
* Talk to friends who eat this way to get practical, hands-on advice.
* Contact the UK Vegetarian Society (see page 269), for information, advice and support.

Common pitfalls

When attempting to feed your child a vegetarian diet:

* Make only moderate use of cheese. Although a good source of calcium and protein, it is also high in saturated fat and salt.
* Limit the use of highly-processed and ready-made foods. They may be vegetarian, but they could still be high in added sugar, salt, unhealthy fats or additives. Instead, learn to cook from fresh.
* Learn to read labels. 'Natural', 'Healthy' or 'Good-For-You' labels do not guarantee a vegetarian product. Many foods you would never suspect to include animal derivatives do in fact contain them.
* Don't run before you can walk. Learning to cook and eat vegetarian is like learning a new language; it takes time to reach proficiency.

There is more than one way to eat, just as there is more than one way to speak, dress and learn. If your child shows vegetarian tendencies, accept the challenge with grace – it may well benefit the entire family.

Vegetarian dishes are not the preserve of vegetarians. A mainly plant-based diet is suitable for everyone, and I have included several meat-free recipes which can be enjoyed by vegetarians and non-vegetarians alike.

Recipes suitable for vegetarians:

Tagliatelle with Lemon and Courgette Sauce (page 191)
Creamy Vegetarian Lasagne (page 200)
Vegetarian Rice (page 206)
The Best Macaroni Cheese (page 207)
Baked Barley Risotto (page 212)
Roasted Red Pepper and Feta Frittata (page 167)
Chickpeas in Tomato Sauce (page 164)
Green Monster Pasta (page 173)
Roasted Vegetables with Couscous (page 174)
Hearty Bean Soup (page 180)
Jungle Soup (page 171)
Carrot, Lentil and Sweet Potato Soup (page 187)
Sweetcorn Chowder (page 186)
Homemade Pesto (page 184)
All snacks and baking/pudding recipes (pages 215–31)

Feeding During Illness

When children fall ill, especially if a fever is involved, their instinctive reaction is to withdraw from the world, reject food and drink and to sleep it out. As a parent you might become anxious – high fever, no food – but it is, in fact, a perfectly healthy response. Limiting food intake and activity helps the immune system focus on the goal in hand: fighting and eliminating the invader – a bacteria or virus.

Do not force or tempt your child to eat if he has no desire for food. Give him the time to be ill, under strict supervision, of course. Children tend to be more in tune with their bodies than adults, and a normally healthy child can go a day or two without solid food intake so long as he continues to take in fluids. You need to judge for yourself whether the lack of appetite is truly a result of the acute illness, or the manipulative behaviour of a fussy eater. In the former case, the loss of appetite is natural and should be supported with fluids as above. In the latter, you are dealing with the extension of a routine problem. (See 'Food Fussiness' on page 118 for ways to deal with this.)

The most important thing you can do when a child is ill is to ensure fluid intake so as to avoid dehydration.

* Plain, preferably filtered, water is essential. Often this is the only thing children desire when they are unwell. Leave a bottle of water near your child's bed so that he can help himself when you are not around. Offer little sips frequently, but let him decide how much he can take in one go.
* If your child is vomiting or has diarrhoea then you will also need to replace lost salts through the use of oral rehydration solutions. Encourage them to drink this rather than water or juices. Buy the commercial

packets rather than making your own as it is very easy to cause an imbalance in salt levels which can be life threatening.

* A beaker or a straw can make drinking easier.
* In general, fluids should be warm or at room temperature.
* Diluted fruit or vegetable juices, preferably fresh and organic, are nourishing and easily digestible. Choose simple, fairly neutral fruit and vegetables, such as apple, pear and carrot.
* Herbal teas, such as camomile, cinnamon or vitamin-C-rich lemon or rosehip can also help. Tea can be sweetened with a little honey, if desired.
* A warm broth (see recipe on page 94) is very soothing; chicken soup has been the classic remedy for colds and flu for generations.

Vitamin C

Many parents consider giving their child vitamin C supplements if they are experiencing frequent colds. Be sure to discuss any supplements with your child's doctor before giving them, and ensure that you only give the dose they recommend. Don't forget to encourage plenty of rest and sleep.

Your child may only be able to take a few sips at a time. When your child is acutely ill, give him the broth liquid only. When convalescing, he can eat some of the soup's solids to regain energy. When the acute illness subsides and your child regains some of his energy, his appetite will come back, too. At times children may become ravenous, having in effect fasted for a day or two. This is the time to reintroduce solid foods, preferably lightly cooked vegetables and whole grains. Again, let your child decide how much (or little) he wants to take in; bear in mind he is still not completely well. A fruit-laden, dairy-free fruit smoothie with some ground nuts added (if appropriate) is a good health booster. Thick vegetable soups are nourishing and easy to swallow. Oat or rice porridge is light yet filling. You could use the remains of the clear broth and let the child dip some wholemeal bread into it. Small amounts of fish and chicken can also be added. It is advisable to avoid most dairy foods until your child is completely well, as in my experience they tend to produce phlegm. Live yoghurt is a good food for convalescents, however, as the bacteria in it replace those that may have been depleted during the illness and help to strengthen the immune system. Avoid highly-processed foods, as they contribute few nutrients. The key is to stick to pure, simple, nourishing foods until your child is back on track.

If your child has been waking in the night requiring fluids during his illness, this may continue out of habit after he has recovered. It may take two to three weeks, or longer, for your child to regain his appetite. If, after this time, you are concerned that he still isn't eating properly, keep a food diary for a few days and discuss your concerns with your GP or health visitor. Once you are certain that your child has regained his appetite, he should be drinking enough and eating sufficient quantities of energy-rich foods during the day to ensure that there is no need for supplements during the night. Use your usual routines to encourage your child to settle himself again during the night.

Soup to nourish

When children are unwell and have lost their appetite, a bit of soup can be just the right thing. Here's a recipe for a soup that I find is a comforting remedy. It is clear, fat-free, with plenty of vegetables (organic, if possible). If fish, chicken or meat is to be used in the stock, these should preferably be organic, too.

Basic Chicken Broth for the Ill and Convalescing
* about 1 kg (2 ¼ lb) chicken pieces, preferably organic
* 1 medium onion, quartered
* 1 celery stick with leaves, in 2 cm pieces
* 1 large carrot, in thick chunks
* 1 small sweet potato, in chunks
* 3 bay leaves
* a good handful of parsley and dill
* a few peppercorns
Place all the ingredients in a large pot and add enough water to cover everything by 7–8 cm (3–4 in). Bring to a light boil, then simmer for 2 hours, covered, skimming off any surface froth. Cool, strain and set the meat and vegetables aside for use if desired and appropriate.

Chapter 3

Mealtimes
Made Easy

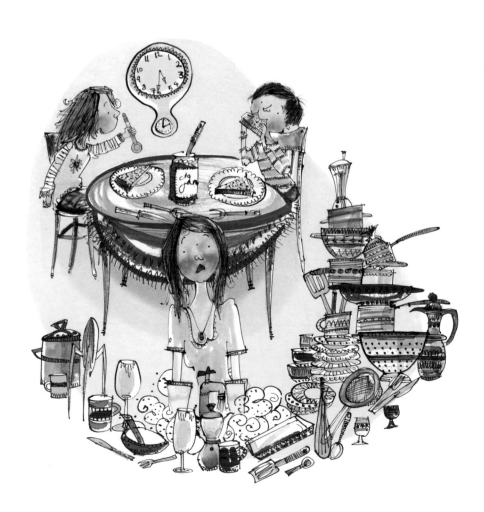

Breakfast

It is widely accepted that breakfast is the most important meal of the day, but it can still be hard for busy parents to find time to plan, prepare and feed a nutritious breakfast to distracted children.

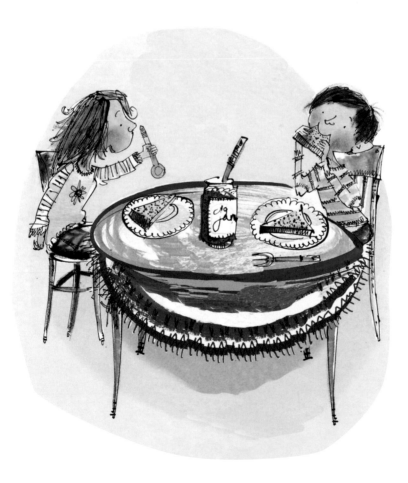

It is vital to lay good foundations of healthy eating, so always ensure that you and your child sit and eat breakfast together. You will be giving your child the best example if you sit down and eat a bowl of muesli with milk, rather than eating a piece of toast as you dash round the kitchen. Not only are you instilling in him the importance of sitting at the table together and eating a nutritious breakfast, but I also believe that your body will be able to more easily digest the food than if you are eating on the go.

> *Research shows that adults and children who eat breakfast are less likely to be overweight than those who skip this essential meal.*

Your child is far more likely to enjoy his breakfast if he can see that you do, too, so prepare foods which you both enjoy and will give you sufficient energy for the morning ahead.

I am a firm believer in the enormous benefits of oat porridge for breakfast. This can be prepared for all the family, and is generally enjoyed by babies from the age of six months – particularly with the addition of a little mashed banana to sweeten it. Older children may like to add a handful of raisins or a little honey or maple syrup to drizzle over it. Warm or cold milk can also be added when serving.

Oats provide an excellent start to the day as they are a complex carbohydrate, giving slow-release energy to power you throughout the morning. They are a great source of dietary fibre, protein, several B vitamins and iron, and are also thought to lower cholesterol, so I would encourage everyone to include oats in their children's diets wherever possible.

Gina's perfect porridge

MAKES ENOUGH FOR ONE ADULT OR TWO CHILDREN
40 g (2 oz) rolled oats
250 ml (8 fl oz) milk (or half milk, half water)

Combine the oats and milk in a saucepan and place over a medium heat. Bring to the boil, stirring, then reduce the heat and allow porridge to simmer, stirring occasionally to prevent sticking, for a few minutes until thickened.

To give you more time in the morning, soak the porridge oats in milk or water (or a combination–my favourite) the night before and pop the mixture into the fridge. This allows the oats to absorb the liquid and cook quickly in the morning.

Breakfast bonus points

* Choose wholegrain cereals that are low in added salt and sugar, such as Weetabix. Serve with milk and perhaps a spoonful of natural yoghurt.
* Try to include some fruit with your breakfast: a handful of dried fruit, fresh berries or chopped fruit on your cereal or with natural yoghurt; or slices of bananas on wholegrain toast.
* If your family struggle to eat their 'five-a-day', pour everyone a glass of fruit juice to enjoy with breakfast. A small glass of pure juice counts as one portion of your daily fruit and vegetable requirements. Fresh juice has far more nutritional value than cartons of processed juice made from concentrate. When buying juice, choose those from the chiller cabinet, if possible.
* Serve fresh fruit smoothies (see page 104) alongside cereal to children who are slow eaters. This way they will enjoy the benefits of all that fruit, in one easy-to-drink glassful.

Breakfast ideas

* oat porridge (see opposite) with a handful of raisins
* wholegrain cereal with milk, sprinkled with fresh berries in season
* homemade muesli (see below) with milk
* natural yoghurt and chopped fresh fruit
* wholegrain toast spread with a little butter and sliced banana
* scrambled eggs and wholegrain toast
* Oaty Breakfast Pancakes (see page 215) with natural yoghurt and fruit purée
* crumpet or muffin topped with a poached egg
* American Eggy Bread (see page 169) with fruit purée

Make your own muesli

To prepare your own tailor-made muesli, combine any of the ingredients below, according to taste. To serve, add grated apple and milk to a small bowlful and refrigerate overnight. Enjoy the softened muesli with extra milk or yoghurt if desired.

rolled oats
wheat flakes
barley flakes
rye flakes
dried fruit: raisins, currants, chopped
apricots, dates, prunes, figs
chopped nuts: walnuts, almonds,
brazil nuts, hazelnuts, pecans, cashews
seeds: sunflower, pumpkin, sesame, flax (also known as linseeds)

When choosing milk to serve with cereal, remember that children under the age of two should have whole milk (preferably organic). Children of two years old and above may have semi-skimmed milk, but do not serve skimmed milk to children under five.

Weekends

This may be a time when the whole family can enjoy breakfast together. You might like to prepare some more time-consuming dishes, such as scrambled egg with smoked salmon and toasted bagels, or homemade pancakes (see page 215) for a brunch-style breakfast. Enjoy the relaxed time together and discuss your plans for the weekend. Don't worry if your baby is throwing toast on the floor – he will learn by watching the rest of the family, sitting happily together.

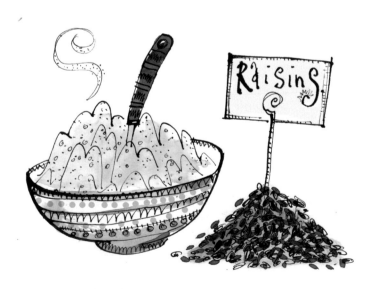

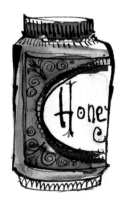

Snacks

Small children are bundles of energy and need constant fuel to keep them going. Between the ages of two and five, children are extremely active and, for some, sitting still long enough to finish a meal is a rare occurrence.

Those who will sit and eat can still only manage small portions at this age. So, in addition to three nutritious meals a day, your child will require little snacks. I find this helps to maintain blood sugar levels (which in turn keep his mood in balance) and hence keep up his energy.

It can be very easy to get into bad habits concerning snacks, either with the timing of them, or the type of foods given. The temptation to give in to your child's requests for the brightly packaged crisps, sweets and sugary drinks can be very strong, particularly if you are away from home and this is the easiest option. Unfortunately, this is also the most inappropriate response, particularly if done regularly. It pays dividends to be prepared for hunger attacks by carrying a supply of suitable snacks to offer your child when you are out. For emergency situations, why not keep a couple of little boxes of raisins in your bag, along with a sachet of oatcakes and a small bottle of water. Get into the habit of popping a banana and an apple into your bag as you leave the house, and you will always have something nutritious to offer your child.

Giving snacks at the same time every day will help to get your child into a routine and he will accept the snacks as mini-meals, and not as extras that he can demand at any time of day. Snacks should be given midway between meals, so that they don't take the edge off a child's appetite. For this reason, snacks should not be too filling but just enough to keep up a child's energy. If a meal is not eaten and a filling snack is offered or demanded close to the next meal, children are unlikely to have much appetite for the meal, and this can lead to a vicious circle of refusing meals and only eating the snacks in-between. This is not so problematic if the snacks offered are nutritious foods such as yoghurt, fruit or sandwiches, but if a habit is formed for processed snacks such as crisps or biscuits, then your child may miss out on essential nutrients.

Avoid giving sugary biscuits as these generally do not provide long-lasting energy. As well as large amounts of sugar, they provide empty calories, filling up your child without providing any goodness. Similarly, avoid savoury snacks such as crisps and highly salted biscuits, as these are full of fat and have little nutritional value.

Fruit and vegetables

Chopped fresh fruit, a handful of dried fruit, or raw chopped vegetables, such as carrots, cucumbers and peppers, are ideal snacks, and will also go some way to ensure your child is getting his five portions of fruit and vegetables a day.

Easy-to-eat fruit

Prepare fruit and vegetables so that they can be held and eaten comfortably. Remember that children, like adults, are lazy when it comes to preparing food and will more happily pick up a biscuit than a whole apple. Cut apples into slices; peel and divide a satsuma into segments. Grapes make a delicious snack, although beware of choking in the younger child. Have a bowl of cut-up fruit in the fridge so that everyone in the family is tempted to snack on it when they are looking for something tasty to eat.

Nuts and seeds

A handful of unsalted nuts, such as walnuts, almonds, cashews or shelled pistachios, mixed with raisins, is a great, healthy, energy-giving snack. However, to avoid the risk of choking, don't offer whole or chopped nuts to children until the age of five. Toasted pumpkin and sunflower seeds also make a nutritious treat for children though I recommend you wait until they are over the age of five (again, due to the risk of choking). Dry-fry them for a minute or two, stirring occasionally to avoid burning. Cool on a plate and store in an airtight container for up to two weeks.

Note that if there any history of allergy in your family then do not offer any nut product before the age of three.

Dip tips

* Serve batons of raw vegetables with homemade dips (see pages 220–1). Arrange a selection of different colours and shapes in an attractive pattern on a plate and encourage your child to try them all.
* Dips such as hummus and avocado guacamole are powerhouses of concentrated energy, and, as well as being great for hungry toddlers, are also perfect for nursing mothers and busy fathers. Note that if your child has a sesame seed allergy you should not offer him commercially-made hummus as it contains sesame seed paste (tahini).
* Prepare a batch of vegetables and store in plastic bags or boxes in the fridge, so that when you settle down to feed the baby, for example, you and your toddler can enjoy a healthy, nutrient-rich snack together.
* Seeing you enjoy the dips should persuade even the most reluctant toddler to try them. If vegetables aren't popular, you could provide breadsticks, rye sticks (see page 219), strips of toasted pitta bread, or even wholemeal toast fingers alongside the dip.
* Chunks of fruit are great to dunk in yoghurt, fruit purée or fromage frais.
* Soak dried apricots, and stew until soft. Purée with a little of the soaking liquid until smooth. This is also excellent stirred into natural yoghurt.

Smoothies and juices

If your child is wary of certain fruit textures, smoothies and fresh juices are a healthy and delicious way of encouraging your child to eat a wide range and quantity of fruits. Juicers and liquidisers can be quite expensive items but, in my opinion they are worth the initial outlay, as once you have started juicing and liquidising, you will find your machine in constant use. If you have been making homemade purées for your baby then you probably already use a food processor or liquidiser.

To make a smoothie, process your chosen soft fruit, washed, peeled and chopped, until combined. The consistency of the smoothie will depend on the fruit you use. You will need to add up to 125 ml (½ pint) of milk, yoghurt or pure fruit juice to give the desired consistency. Juicy fruit will require less liquid, whereas fruit such as bananas and avocado will need more. Experiment with different fruits and liquid to create the taste and texture your child enjoys.

Good fruit combinations to try are:

* 1 banana and ½ a mango
* 1 banana and a handful of strawberries
* 1 banana and ½ an avocado
* 1 banana and a handful of raspberries
* 1 kiwi and a handful of strawberries
* ½ a mango and a handful of strawberries
* 1 peach, 1 apricot and 1 banana
* 1 banana, a handful of raspberries and blueberries
* 1 banana and a small handful of dried apricots (soaked in apple juice overnight)
* 1 banana and a small handful of dried prunes (soaked in apple juice overnight)

Quantities for smoothies depend on personal taste and appetite, so you may want to adjust these to suit you and your child's personal taste.

To make fresh fruit juice, you will need a citrus press or a juicing machine. Fresh juices are packed with vitamins so are worth the effort, although you do need a lot of fruit to make a glass of juice.

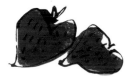

Homemade muffins

* Get into the habit of making and freezing snacks such as muffins in batches. (See pages 216, 216 and 227.) Individual muffins can be defrosted in a matter of minutes and will keep for up to three months in a freezer.

* Homemade muffins can be packed full of energy-giving ingredients, and are far removed from sugary, shop-bought versions.

* Once you have started making muffins, you can add ingredients you know your child will enjoy. Try 50–100 g (2–4 oz) of all kinds of chopped dried fruit (apricots, dates, figs, raisins, cranberries), fresh berries such as blueberries, raspberries and blackcurrants (but not strawberries, which will make the muffins soggy, due to their high water content), grated apple, carrot, courgette and even parsnip.

* Add 50 g (2 oz) of chopped nuts if your child is old enough and doesn't have a nut allergy. Whizz nuts such as walnuts, hazelnuts, pecans, almonds and brazil nuts in a food processor or chop finely by hand, and children will hardly know they are eating them.

For a treat, mix a heaped tablespoon of finely chopped nuts with a scant tablespoon of muscovado sugar and a teaspoon of cinnamon, and sprinkle on muffins before they go in the oven for a delicious, crunchy topping.

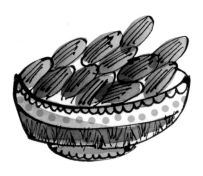

Substantial snacks

At times your child will need something more filling than just fruit or vegetables as a mid-morning snack, particularly if you feel he didn't have an adequate breakfast. Try to include snacks that are not wheat based, as your child is likely to be enjoying foods containing wheat, in the form of pasta, couscous, pastry, pancakes or bread, at mealtimes.

There are lots of tasty wheat-free alternatives available, such as rice cakes, corncakes, oatcakes and rye crackers. These can be served plain or spread with a small amount of butter, fruit spread, cream cheese, or nut butters – try almond as well as peanut, if your child is old enough and doesn't have a nut allergy. For alternative wheat-based snacks try malt loaf, fruit or cheese scones, wheat crackers, brioche rolls and fruit bread. Malt loaf is lower in fat and sugar than other cakes.

Miniature foods are always appealing. Look out for small paper cases to make mini-muffins.

After-school snacks

Children at school can become dehydrated, as drinking is neglected in favour of playing, so, in addition to a snack such as a muffin, offer your wilting schoolchild a drink of water, milk or diluted fruit juice, along with a plate of chopped fruit. This will provide plenty of energy to carry him through homework, after-school activities or playtime with a friend. Alternative after-school snacks include flapjacks (see page 217), oatcakes (see page 222), Scotch pancakes or any of the savoury dips (see page 220–1) served with breadsticks or rice cakes. If it is a hot summer's day, you could offer a homemade smoothie ice lolly.

Yoghurt makes a great snack and is enjoyed by most children, but try to avoid those with lots of additives – sugar, sweeteners, colouring and artificial flavourings. Buy natural yoghurt and add your own flavourings – fruit purée, pure fruit spreads or chopped fruit.

Soups

You don't need to stretch your culinary skills, break the bank or spend hours cooking if you choose to make soup. Your family will eat healthily and deliciously because soup is infinitely versatile and can be adapted to individual tastes.

If your child is reluctant to eat vegetables, soup is a perfect way to hide onions, garlic, leeks, sweet potato or carrot, blended into a smooth, easy-to-eat concoction. A thick soup is ideal for toddlers just learning to wield a spoon, as well as being a perfect purée for a weaning baby. Remember to leave out any seasoning if you are planning to use the soup as a baby purée.

Stock

The basis of soup is a good stock. A homemade stock is ideal, but don't dismiss the reduced-salt brands of stock and bouillon available in powder or concentrate.

* After Sunday lunch, put your chicken carcase into a stock pot or large saucepan with an onion, a couple of roughly chopped carrots and sticks of celery, some stems of parsley, sprigs of thyme, a bay leaf and a few black peppercorns, and perhaps a couple of cloves if you have them. Cover with water and bring to the boil, then reduce to a low simmer for a couple of hours.
* The same method applies to fish stock but it should not be cooked for longer than 30 minutes or it will be bitter. You may also add fennel to fish stock for extra flavour. Your fishmonger will usually give you fish heads and bones for free.
* For vegetable stock, replace the chicken or fish with a few more vegetables and cook for an hour.
* Cool, refrigerate and skim off any fat.
* Stock freezes well – store it in your freezer for up to two months.

Quick and easy soups

With a tub of reduced-salt bouillon in the cupboard and some dried, frozen or tinned vegetables, serving up a wholesome soup is only minutes away.

* Cook frozen peas in stock until soft (about ten minutes), and blend them, perhaps with a tin of flageolet beans to add earthiness to the sweetness.
* Simmer a handful of red lentils in bouillon for half an hour. Then they won't need to be blended.
* Any frozen vegetables can be cooked in stock with pasta and served as a chunky soup with some grated cheese on top.

Garnishes

Children love adding their own garnishes at the table. The following might add protein or simply spice up a simple soup:

* grated cheese or a swirl of yoghurt or cream
* croutons – cubes of bread tossed in a tablespoon of olive oil and baked in a hot oven for ten minutes
* pieces of fried bacon or mild chorizo
* chopped fresh herbs – coriander, parsley and chervil
* a squeeze of lemon juice is particularly good with earthy soups such as lentil
* hunks of crusty bread, warm from the oven

Useful soup tips

Thick or thin, smooth or chunky, homemade soup is infinitely adaptable.

* A hand-held blender which you plunge into the pan saves the messy business of pouring the soup into a food processor and back. It also allows you to control the level of blending. Some children adore a velvety-smooth soup; others prefer recognisable pieces of vegetable.
* Consider setting aside chunks of vegetables or meat to add after the soup has been blended.
* Use potatoes, rice, split red lentils, pearl barley, millet flakes or pasta to thicken soup rather than flour.
* If adding milk or cream, let the soup cool slightly to avoid curdling. Use sparingly or the dairy products will dominate.

* For the child who likes to know exactly what he's eating, Japanese-style soups are perfect. See the recipe for Chicken Noodle Soup on page 181.

Soup recipes:

Hearty Bean Soup (page 180)
Jungle Soup (page 171)
Carrot, Lentil and Sweet Potato Soup (page 187)
Sweetcorn Chowder (page 186)
Chicken Noodle Soup (page 181)

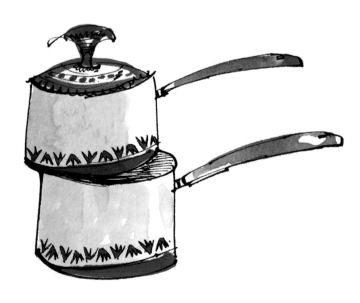

Salads

Young children can be wary of salads, but if introduced carefully, they can become lifelong favourites, with the huge health benefits of vitamin-rich vegetables.

Some children are suspicious of dishes where everything is mixed together, so why not serve the salad ingredients in individual bowls and allow children to create their own salad with a choice of vegetables and other ingredients. Older children could be encouraged to include at least two different coloured ingredients, whereas very small children should be praised for trying even one new item.

* Make salads visually appealing by cutting vegetables into different shapes and including a variety of colours and textures. Try shaving courgette curls with a potato peeler, grating carrot, or cutting long strips of red pepper.
* Include fruit with vegetables to make sweet and sour salads. Melon balls are fun, thirst-quenching and work with a variety of vegetables.
* Dried fruit is a popular addition in salads.
* Some vegetables normally served cooked are also great in salads and retain all their nutrients when served raw. Try small florets of cauliflower, broccoli, baby sweetcorn, mangetout and sugarsnap peas.
* Include pulses in salads. Tinned pulses are very convenient as they only need draining and rinsing before use.

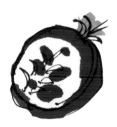

Dressings

Offer dressings separately, as some children prefer salad undressed. In addition, dressings can be too strong for children, so try some sweeter, child-friendly ones, such as:

* 3 tbsp olive oil, 1 tbsp fresh lemon juice and 1 tsp honey. Adding chopped fresh herbs – basil or oregano, for example – is a super way to introduce children to the pleasures of green-flecked foods.
* 3 tbsp olive oil, 1 tbsp reduced-salt soya sauce, 1 tbsp fresh orange juice and 1 tsp runny honey.

Mix the dressing in a jar with a screw-top lid and it will last for two to three weeks. Add a whole clove of garlic to the jar for a gentle garlic flavour.

Super salads

The following salad ideas can all be served with or without dressing. If you prefer your salad undressed, you may need to add some fresh lemon juice to prevent browning on apples, pears and avocado.

* grated carrot, grated apple, raisins and poppy seeds with lemony dressing (see above)
* halved cherry tomatoes, avocado chunks, cubes of mozzarella, torn fresh basil leaves
* halved, cooked French beans, cooked peas, chopped and seeded tomato
* cooked brown rice, thinly sliced apple, and raisins
* sliced pear, avocado chunks and walnut
* cucumber cubes and finely chopped dill
* baby spinach leaves and chunks of orange
* baby new potatoes, chopped egg, halved cherry tomatoes and chives
* finely sliced white cabbage, grated carrot and sunflower seeds
* red kidney beans with French beans and tomatoes
* butter beans with tuna and chopped cucumber

Salad toppers

Seeds are highly nutritious. Pumpkin and sunflower seeds are a good source of protein and minerals. To make them deliciously nutty, dry-fry carefully for a minute or two over a gentle heat, stirring occasionally to prevent burning.

Sprinkle on salads when cool and store the remainder in an airtight container for future use. Sesame seeds are also good for you, providing protein and calcium. Sesame is a potential allergen, however, so do not give to children under the age of three if there is a history of allergy in the family.

Nuts are also great to include in salads, as they are powerhouses of nutrition. Again, take care if your family has a history of allergy. Walnuts are a good source of omega-3 and combine well with apple, avocado, raisin and grated carrot. Cashew nuts are also rich in protein and minerals and are often popular with children as they are quite sweet and soft. Do remember that it is not advisable to give whole or chopped nuts to children under the age of five due to the risk of choking.

Raisins work well in salads, providing sweetness as well as antioxidants. They are particularly good with crunchy apples, grated carrots and finely sliced white cabbage.

Olives can be popular with children and provide a nice savoury taste. Make sure the stones have been removed before offering them to your child. Although rich in 'good' mono-unsaturated fats, olives are very salty and should be enjoyed in small amounts.

Top tip

Children love to eat food they have grown. Sprinkle some mustard or cress seeds on a few sheets of damp, folded kitchen paper on a plate, and place it on a sunny windowsill. Keep the paper damp (but not waterlogged) and after four or five days you will have some delicious sprouted mustard or cress to add to your salads or sandwiches.

Crunchy crumbs made from freshly made and blitzed wholemeal breadcrumbs, baked for ten minutes in a medium-hot oven, can be sprinkled on salads to provide texture and fibre.

Top Tip

Remember, fruit and vegetables lose some of their vitamins once cut and exposed to the atmosphere, so try not to make salads too far in advance of eating them.

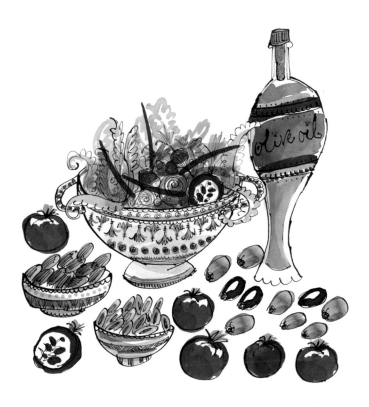

Family Meals

Sitting down to a family meal at the end of the day used to be a daily ritual that was taken for granted. These days, however, it is the exception rather than the rule.

Two out of three British families no longer share most of their dinners, and, sadly, many families prefer eating their ready-made, supermarket meals in front of the television. In an ironic twist, families are too busy watching food programmes on the television to enjoy a shared, home-cooked meal!

However, a shared meal should not be idealised. At times the children can bicker, whine and fuss over food; the adults may be stressed from a long and busy day; and the food may not necessarily be healthy. Nevertheless, the statistics are clear: children who regularly eat with their parents are healthier, happier and do better at school. Psychological studies also show that the real benefits of shared family meals become apparent when the children are teenagers. The more often families eat together, the less likely children are to smoke, drink, take drugs, get depressed, develop eating disorders and consider suicide.

Obviously, the way we eat has as much of an effect on our health and well-being as the nutrients we take in. Good nutrition is not just about vitamins, minerals, antioxidants and healthy fats. It is also about the other types of nutrition a shared meal provides: physical, social, emotional and educational.

Nutritionally speaking, as a parent you stand a much greater chance of instilling healthy eating habits in your children if you share the same table with them and lead by example. Sitting with your children and eating a healthy meal together is the best way to get the message across. Cooking a fresh, homemade, nutritious dinner may take more time, but children fed in this way are less likely to become obese or snack on unhealthy processed foods. They learn first hand, day in, day out, what a proper meal consists of, and lessons learned in childhood last for life.

Table manners

Socially, the family meal is the best time to teach your children table manners. With fast food and snacking-on-the-go, eating with our hands has almost become the norm, and many children do not know how to handle a knife and a fork properly. The family table is a safe environment in which to learn and practise dining skills before venturing out to the world. More than just filling their tummies, a meal is about civilising children and teaching them the ways of your culture, of which eating is a central one. As with any other skill you wish to master, doing it regularly, routinely and reliably will get results.

The family dinner time is also a good moment for children to learn about sharing and compromise. Many parents make the mistake of catering separately to a child's individual preferences or cook 'kiddie meals'. By preparing one-meal-for-all you send out a clear and powerful message to your child: you can't always have it your way. Not only that: we as a family are in it together, like it or not. Practically speaking, a one-meal-for-all also makes sense for busy parents, cuts down on the work and has the potential to be more nutritious; you might cook one healthy meal, but you wouldn't cook three separate ones.

At the dinner table your child will learn to practise restraint. He will have to wait for others to start eating, or stay at the table until everyone has finished. He will need to consider others when taking his portion. Modern children expect – and usually get – immediate gratification, so learning a measure of restraint is good for them. The same holds true for routine. Sitting together often enough in the same place at (roughly) the same time instils a sense of security and regularity. It conveys the wisdom that there is a time and place for everything, even when everyone is busy rushing off in different directions at different times. The family dinner can serve as the day's anchor.

Practically speaking, a family meal counts as one even if Mum or Dad are not present. It's the regular, reliable ritual that matters. Absence of one of the parents during the week will make family weekend dinners even more special.

During the meal switch off the television, and let the phone go unanswered. This may be the only quiet time you have as a family, so make the most of it.

Preparing family meals

To cut down on last-minute, stressful cooking:

* Keep it simple. Offer good, nutritious meals not gourmet fare. Children like unfussy food. Reserve experimentation with chefs' recipes for the weekend.
* Prepare ahead: make a quick dish and leave it in the oven or slow cooker with the timer set for the evening.
* Do some planning at the weekend, especially if you are out at work during the week. Decide what you'll make during the week and shop for the ingredients at the weekend.
* Keep a good selection of different sauces on hand; they can turn basic ingredients into culinary delights.
* Write down and pin up in the kitchen a list of favourite dishes that you know are quick, easy and preferably nutritious; curries, stir fries and meal-in-a-bowl soups are all possibilities. Resort to the list when you run out of ideas.
* Ask for help if you need it. Children of all ages love helping out in the kitchen, and you may be surprised how useful they can actually be. Learn to think of your children as your meal task force. They'll happily measure, chop, mix, wash and arrange, according to their age and ability. If you want them out of the kitchen area, get them to set the table. The more you involve them, the more they'll learn helpful skills and a measure of responsibility.

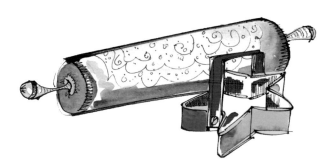

Food Fussiness

Fussy eaters are on the increase in this era of almost unlimited choice and availability in terms of food, and it sometimes seems that the more choice you give children, the more they refuse to eat. Often, they will reject the nourishing meal you have painstakingly prepared but will happily eat over-processed, fatty, salty foods.

Many children become fussy eaters at some time in their lives and, be comforted, most outgrow it. The problem usually arises between the ages of one and five years when the child is learning to take control of his behaviour and to exercise choice and will.

Prevention
* Start taking measures against future fussy eating when your child is young. Children who are weaned appropriately on a varied diet are less likely to become fussy. Offer small quantities of different foods to your baby rather than large amounts of one or two foods. From around nine months your baby becomes aware of different colours and shapes, try to make food look attractive. A selection of two or three different-coloured vegetables served with fish or chicken will be more appealing than a mush.
* Whatever the situation, don't use food as a reward or punishment. Saying, 'If you don't eat your greens, you can't have any pudding' immediately communicates to the child that greens are a punishment and pudding is a reward.
* Don't lose sight of the fact that children usually grow out of fussy eating and that it is unlikely to have any damaging long-term consequences.
* Your anxiety can have the effect of discouraging your child from eating. He starts to associate food with negative feelings or thoughts and the situation can go from bad to worse. Meals must be happy times.

* Don't let your child fill up with snacks and drinks before meals.
* At mealtimes, it is best to let your child eat at least half his food before offering water. If he must have fruit juice, make sure it is well diluted.
* If your child refuses a meal, don't offer substitute snacks.
* Try to stick to regular mealtimes and avoid distractions such as television.
* Never force-feed your child. It can be extremely distressing to all concerned and lead to extreme food aversion.

Dealing with fussy eaters

* If your toddler is getting fussy and refusing food, try serving very small portions on a larger plate. Give him lots of praise when he eats it all. Gradually increase the portion by a tiny amount every three or four days until he starts eating normally again.
* Once your child is able to eat bite-sized pieces of solid food, stop preparing separate meals and introduce family foods as soon as possible. Most things you prepare will be suitable for your baby, providing you don't add salt. It is too easy to fall into the trap of only serving foods you know your children will eat.
* Allow your child to taste things from your plate. Someone else's food often looks more tempting than what is in front of him.
* Whenever possible, eat as a family and make sure you set a good example with your own eating habits. Invite other children whom you know to be good eaters.
* If your child refuses to eat a particular food, try not to get upset, and be aware that a lecture will probably go in one ear and out the other. Simply remove the plate quietly and try again another day. If you don't respond, it is quite probable that your child will get bored with his own behaviour.
* Don't introduce new foods all the time. Concentrate on what your child will eat and gradually build on these, possibly introducing a new food that is related to one he already likes. For instance, if he likes bread but not eggs, try making American Eggy Bread (see page 169). If he refuses fruit but likes ice cream, try serving them together. He will probably try some of the fruit.
* Praise your child when he tries new foods.

* Keep mealtimes short and don't sit there battling over one mouthful. If you eat and chat, it is quite likely that your child will do the same and eat without thinking about it.
* From the age of about four, allow your child to serve himself from dishes on the table to enable him to exercise choice.

Top tip

If your child won't eat cooked vegetables, offer them raw as crudités, which children often prefer. Cut them into bite-sized pieces and serve with a familiar dip such as hummus. Simply place them on a table where your child spends time and see what happens. The sweetness of carrots is appealing and you can try filling the groove of celery sticks with cream cheese or peanut butter.

At your wits' end?

If you have tried everything you can think of but your child still refuses to eat anything healthy that is placed in front of him, there are still a few things you can do.

* The first step is to get your child's health and development checked. Get him weighed and measured and ask for a blood test to check his iron levels.
* If his diet has been unbalanced, your GP will be able to advise whether to give him a vitamin and mineral supplement. Remember that this is a temporary solution – supplements cannot replace the nutrition reaped from fresh foods.
* Once you're reassured that he is well, you can follow the advice in the box on the opposite page.

Ending the Battle

* Stress is an appetite-killer for many people, including children. If your child knows that a battle is about to start when he sits at the table, his stress levels rise, releasing hormones which reduce the blood supply to the stomach which may lessen his appetite. So the first thing to do is to call a truce. Make sure everyone at the table is aware of, and in agreement about, the changes you are making.

* A refusal to eat vegetables is a common problem, although this system works for any type of food. Using vegetables as an example, the first step is to give them to everyone else at the table but not to the fussy eater. Praise him for what he does eat. Do not discuss your motives or anything relating to this issue. Just serve the vegetables, and act as if nothing has happened. Try to let go of the stress you normally experience at mealtimes.

* Continue this new behaviour for at least one week. Even if your child is still not eating vegetables, mealtimes will have become more relaxed and that is a firm platform to build on.

* The next stage of the strategy is to find a vegetable that your child has never tried or seen. Starting with something sweet like sweet potato or butternut squash is a good idea. Serve it at the table with the rest of the meal but do not offer your fussy child any. While you eat, discuss the vegetable – where it grows, how it looks, anything to make it sound interesting. If you can trigger your child's curiosity, he is more likely to try something new.

* Do not expect your child to try it the first time but continue to introduce new vegetables or prepare familiar ones in new ways. Never offer your child some or even suggest he tries it. Eventually most children will ask for a taste.

* Be consistent and patient. Bad eating habits are often years in the making and will not disappear overnight. Some children can be very stubborn, and it takes a lot of courage and willpower not to give in.

Chapter 4

Cooking
Made Easy

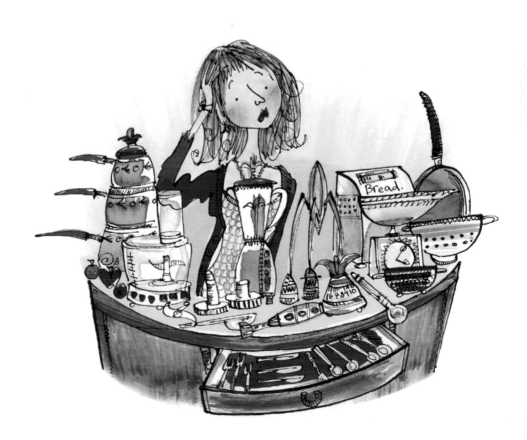

Store Cupboard Basics

Although you will be shopping regularly for fresh ingredients, it is useful to have a supply of some items to hand that you often use. Then, if you suddenly need to rustle up a meal in a hurry, you can relax in the knowledge that you already have the ingredients.

Most of us are fortunate to have access to fresh vegetables and fruit, but there are, in fact, instances where tinned or frozen varieties are preferable.

* Processed tomatoes contain higher quantities than raw tomatoes of the antioxidant lycopene, which some research claims helps to fight against cardiovascular disease, various cancers, diabetes and osteoporosis. So if your child has the occasional dollop of tomato ketchup with his meal, rest assured that it is doing him more benefit than harm.
* Serving cooked tomatoes in a meal containing some fat, though it only needs to be a teaspoon or so, also helps the absorption of lycopene by the body.
* Tinned red salmon is another friend. Whereas much fresh salmon is farmed, tinned salmon is wild, as stated on the label, so you don't need to worry about any chemicals used in production.
* Frozen vegetables such as peas and sweetcorn can be higher in vitamins than their fresh counterparts, as they are frozen immediately after picking, thereby minimising the loss of vitamins.

Although pasta is an ideal store cupboard meal provider, with a handy supply of easy-to-cook grains such as couscous, quinoa and bulghar wheat, you can easily produce a nutritious meal with the addition of steamed or roasted vegetables and perhaps some grated cheese.

Items to keep in stock

Fridge
Butter
Try to use unsalted butter to cut down your salt intake.
Milk
Organic if possible.
Eggs
Free-range or organic.
Mild Cheddar cheese
For children's snacks.
Mature Cheddar cheese
Imparts greater flavour to sauces.
Parmesan cheese
For risottos and pasta dishes.
Natural yoghurt
Use as a healthy breakfast or dessert with fresh fruit and to replace cream in cooking.
Salad
According to season, such as salad leaves, cucumber, avocado, tomatoes.
Vegetables
For crudités, such as carrots, celery, peppers.

Freezer
Frozen peas
Frozen sweetcorn
Pitta bread

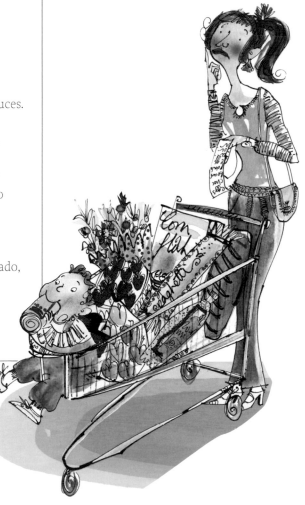

Store Cupboard

Tinned tomatoes

Available whole or chopped and essential for all kinds of dishes, including pasta sauces, soups, pizza sauce, vegetable and meat casseroles.

Passata

A runny tomato paste, useful for tomato-based sauces, soups and casseroles.

Tomato purée

A thick paste of unseasoned concentrate of tomatoes, which provides an intense tomato flavour to soups, sauces and meat-based casseroles.

Tinned fish

Tuna, red salmon, sardines, mackerel and pilchards. Healthy and convenient for sandwiches, and for adding to pasta sauces and salads.

Tinned pulses

Chickpeas, kidney beans, cannellini beans, butter beans and flageolet beans. These are already cooked and require only draining and rinsing before use. Useful for bulking out meat-based sauces, adding to salads, soups and casseroles, and dips such as hummus.

Dried pulses

Very economical. Use just as you would tinned pulses but they require soaking overnight before cooking.

Dried lentils

Including red, brown, green and Puy lentils – easy to cook as they require no soaking and are a wonderful addition to soups, salads and casseroles.

Dried pasta

There are many shapes and sizes available. Choose tiny shapes for soups and for babies, and large shapes for pasta salads. Flat sheets of pasta are used in lasagne and baked dishes.

Egg noodles and rice noodles

Highly versatile and quick to cook. Use for stir fries, soups and salads.

Rice

Brown and white.

Other grains

Quinoa, bulgar wheat, couscous, barley, millet (see page 46).

Rice cakes

Oatcakes

Breakfast cereals

Choose ones with low levels of sugar and salt, such as Weetabix and Shredded Wheat.

Rolled oats

Useful for porridge, oatcakes, flapjacks and crumble toppings.

Dried fruit

Such as raisins, apricots, dates, mango.

Flour

*Use *plain flour* for thickening sauces, making biscuits, pastry and pancakes.

Self-raising flour is used for cakes and sponges. Look for wholemeal self-raising flour for a less refined alternative.

Strong flour – sometimes called bread flour – has a high gluten content and is ideal for making bread and pizza dough. Choose from white or wholemeal, or combine the two for a lighter texture. There are many other flours available which can often be substituted for conventional wheat flour.

Spelt flour is made from an ancient variety of wheat and contains more protein and fat than ordinary wheat. Spelt flour is great for breadmaking and makes delicious pizza dough, biscuits and cakes. As bread made with spelt flour rises more quickly, you will need to reduce the rising time.

Rye flour is a dark, heavy flour with a low gluten content. It makes dense, sticky bread with a characteristic flavour, and can be combined with wheat flour for lighter-textured loaves. Rye flour can also partially replace wheat flour in many cake, biscuit, pancake and scone recipes.

Barley flour is available from health food shops and can be used to partially replace some of the wheat flour in breadmaking. Also useful in biscuits and crumble toppings.

Rice flour can be used like barley flour, but has a denser texture. It makes lovely crunchy cookies and shortbread.

Buckwheat flour is gluten-free and therefore unsuitable for breadmaking, but it has a pleasant sweet flavour and can be added to biscuit and pancake recipes.

Polenta flour—also known as cornmeal or maize flour. This is high in protein and low in fat, and has a beautiful golden colour. It gives a lovely crunchy texture to biscuits and muffins (see Courgette Cornmeal Muffins, page 216).

Raw cane sugar

Choose unrefined sugar if possible as it is a more natural product, having been subjected to less processing.

Honey

Has long been thought of as a natural remedy, and has antiseptic healing properties. It is totally natural and can be used to replace sugar in many recipes but can only be given to children from the age of one. As it is sweeter than sugar you will need to use less. Use honey to sweeten smoothies, porridge, natural yoghurt or spread on wholemeal toast, crumpets and pancakes for an easy, energy-giving breakfast.

Maple syrup

A natural sweetener with a delicious toasty flavour which can be used in the same way as honey.

Oils

Olive oil is a delicious oil containing the healthier mono-unsaturated fats. Olive oils vary according to the success of the olive harvest, the type of olive used and the way it is pressed. Extra-virgin olive oil is the most highly prized and is a result of the first pressing of the olive, however, this oil does not stand up to high heat so use these fine, fruity oils for salad dressings, marinades or for drizzling over lightly cooked vegetables. Other olive oils result from further pressings and may be combined and processed to produce oils lighter in flavour. These are suitable for use in frying, dressings, marinades and baking.

Sunflower oil has little flavour and can be safely heated to high temperatures, so it is a good economical oil for cooking. It can also be used to replace butter in many cake and muffin recipes.

Vegetable oil—look for ones made from rapeseed, as this is a source of omega-3 fatty acids, and so is considered a heart-healthy oil. It is an economical, all-purpose cooking oil. Avoid oils made from saturated fats such as palm oil.

White wine and balsamic vinegar

These vinegars are used in salad dressings and marinades.

This is made by fermenting soya beans, with the addition of salt, water and wheat or barley flour. Use for stir fries and to give flavour to Asian dishes. Look for low-salt varieties and the naturally fermented, wheat-free tamari.

Add these to soups, stocks and stews when you don't have time to make fresh stock. However, they are extremely high in salt so look for reduced-salt varieties and check that they don't contain monosodium glutamate (MSG).

Freezing Food

If you can, I strongly recommend that you buy a freezer, if you don't have one already. If you are still weaning your baby, you will be able to make batches of purées for him that can be frozen in ice cube trays and defrosted individually later. In this way you can take advantage of plentiful supplies of cheap fruit and vegetables when in season to make easy, healthy meals.

Packing food for the freezer

* Make sure cooked food is covered as quickly as possible and transfer it to the freezer as soon as it is cool enough.
* Never put warm food into a fridge or freezer.
* Check the temperature of your freezer on a freezer thermometer. It should read -18 °C. If you don't already have a freezer thermometer they can be bought from good hardware shops or the cookware section in large department stores.
* Never re-freeze cooked food. Food can only be put back into the freezer if it was originally frozen raw then defrosted and cooked. A raw frozen chicken breast, defrosted, for example, can be frozen as a cooked casserole.

* If preparing puréed baby food, using an ice cube tray, fill the tray with puréed food, open-freeze until solid, then pop the cubes out of the tray and into a sterilised plastic box. Non-sterilised items such as plastic bags can be used for babies from the age of six months. Seal well and freeze.

Defrosting tips

* Defrost frozen (covered) food in the fridge overnight or leave at room temperature if you forget, transferring it to the fridge as soon as it has defrosted.
* Make sure food is covered at all times and stand it on a plate to catch any drips.
* Never speed up defrosting by putting food into warm or hot water.
* Always use defrosted food within 24 hours.

Re-heating tips

* When batch cooking, take out the portion of food for use now and freeze the rest as soon as possible. Don't be tempted to re-heat the entire mixture and then freeze what is left.
* Don't be tempted to freeze or re-heat any leftovers from your child's plate, even if he has barely touched his meal. Small children are much more susceptible than adults to food poisoning so get in the habit of throwing leftovers away immediately.
* Re-heat food only once.

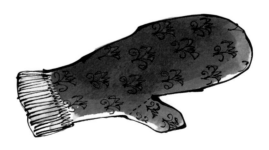

Useful Equipment

If you are going to prepare daily meals for your family, it is worth investing in a few pieces of kitchen equipment to save time and to make your life easier.

Essential items

Once you start weaning your baby you will find a hand-held blender invaluable for making purées. This can blend small quantities at a time, making it extremely convenient for puréeing your baby's portion of a family meal, once he is over nine months old and is enjoying the same foods as the rest of the family. Remember to remove your baby's portion before seasoning food. Hand-held blenders are ideal for puréeing soups in the pan, removing the need to transfer hot soup to a liquidiser. They are also great for puréeing soft fruit for purées and instant desserts. These blenders are small enough to transport, so are vital bits of kit to pack if you are travelling with your baby, either to stay with friends for the weekend or going on holiday. If travelling abroad, don't forget to take an appropriate socket adaptor.

A food processor is extremely useful for puréeing large quantities of food. They are more powerful than hand-held blenders so can cope with more robust foods. They are also useful for chopping nuts and vegetables, for whizzing up dips and pesto as well as making breadcrumbs. Once you have a liquidiser or food processor you will wonder how you managed without one. Food processors are even more versatile, as they have different attachments which can slice, grate and mix cakes and pastry.

Handy items

If you and your family eat a lot of bread then seriously consider buying a breadmaker. It will enable you to make fresh bread daily, using a variety of flours and additional ingredients such as dried fruit, nuts and seeds, without the need for the preservatives and large quantities of salt used in commercial breadmaking. Making bread manually is a fun activity to do with your child occasionally, but if you need to produce large quantities of sandwiches for packed lunches then it is definitely worth buying a breadmaker. They are available at various prices, so you should be able to find one to suit your requirements and budget.

To make the most nutritious and delicious fruit and vegetable juices, a juicer can be invaluable. There may be benefits of fresh juice over heat-treated juice made from fruit concentrate as fresh juice is packed with vitamins, some of which may be lost in processing. Fruit juices can also count as a portion of the recommended five-a-day fruit and vegetables, and are an easy way to encourage children to eat fruit. Children will enjoy experimenting with different fruit and vegetable combinations, and may be encouraged to try new and more unusual ones.

An ice cream maker is a luxury item, but using one can be a great way to enjoy all sorts of soft fruit – particularly if you grow your own fruit and have a glut of it.

Small utensils

* Potato ricer – makes the smoothest mashed potato with ease.
* Rotary whisk – great fun and safe for children to use to help whisk cream and egg whites.
* Round-ended knife – suitable for children to use to chop vegetables and fruit when they are old enough.
* Peeler – find ones that older children can use safely, as they love to help out in the kitchen, peeling carrots and potatoes.
* Small wooden spoons – easier for little hands to hold.
* Small rolling pin – more wieldy for your child to use than an adult-sized one.
* Selection of cookie cutters.

Chapter 5

Cooking
Made Fun

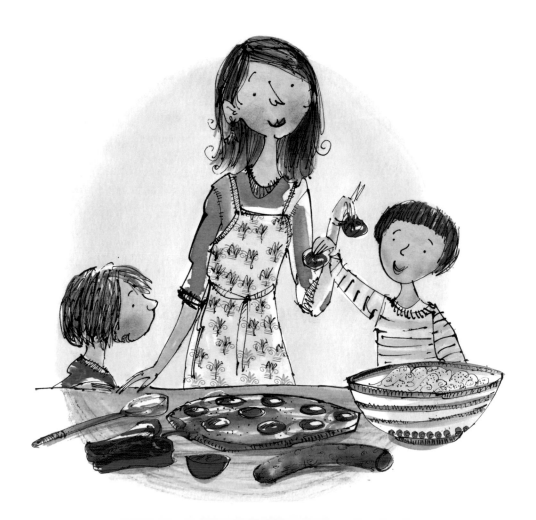

Cooking with Children

I strongly recommend that you involve your child in as many aspects of food preparation as possible from an early age, including choosing foods, shopping, preparation, cooking and washing up.

If your child feels included, not only will he gain a healthy respect for food and where it comes from, he will also avoid fussiness towards food, learn important life skills, and gain in self-confidence as he feels that he is contributing to the daily tasks of the family. Most importantly, this is a creative activity you and your child can share, and you will gain huge pleasure from doing these things together. The look of pride on your child's face when he sees the fruits of his labour cooked and finished so that he is then able to offer them to others to taste, will warm your heart and erase your frustrations when you see the kitchen floor is covered with flour and the table smeared with butter.

Baking with Mum or Dad is one of the greatest pleasures of childhood. There is something so wholesome about the smell of home-baked bread and cookies, and even the smallest child can happily spend time in the kitchen helping in the creation of these delicious items. Very young children can help spoon out and pour the ingredients into the bowl and stir the mixture; older ones will also be able to help measure out ingredients and read the numbers on the scales. This is an ideal opportunity to discuss why some things are heavier than others. The popularity of stirring doesn't diminish as children grow older, and you may find you have to 'ration' everyone's stirs to keep the event fair.

A plate of home-baked cookies can be a delightful gift for grandparents or friends, and your child will experience delight and pride that he has created something which is enjoyed by others.

Making bread

Bread is ideal to make with toddlers, as they are able to knead and play with the dough to their hearts' content with no adverse effects on the ensuing bread. You will just need to watch that they don't eat the dough before it is cooked, as uncooked flour could cause indigestion. As children grow older they can be encouraged to make their pieces of dough into shapes – faces, animals and flowers, or simply balls, snakes or craggy rocks. These can be decorated with raisins before being left to rise. Dough can also be rolled flat with child-sized rolling pins, and then rolled up again into sausage shapes. Both tasks encourage manual dexterity.

Bread is one of the most fundamental parts of our diets, and making bread with children is not only a fun activity; it also teaches them a new skill and gives them a powerful sense of achievement when they see their wonderful, golden-brown loaf of bread taken out of the oven.

Experiment with a variety of flours to make bread, using not only white, but also wholemeal, granary, spelt and rye flours.

Making pizzas

Once you have begun making bread dough, it is a small step to making pizzas. In my experience, this is something that all children like to eat and also to make. Once you have kneaded and played with the dough, and left it to rise, you can roll it out into individual child-sized pizzas. With a base of tomato sauce, children can then choose from a variety of toppings. Choice is a great thing for a child and if he feels comfortable and in control of the situation, your child may choose to try toppings he would normally refuse. (See page 182 for pizza dough recipe and suggested toppings.)

Wholemeal spelt flour in your dough makes a great pizza base. You can use all spelt flour, or half spelt and half strong white flour for a paler crust.

Helping in the kitchen

If you are busy preparing a meal, it can be fun to encourage your child to help you with some of the tasks. Toddlers love to stand at the sink with a bowl of bubbly water and 'do the washing-up'. Show him how to use the brush or sponge and let him wash some plastic utensils for you. Make sure he wears a waterproof apron, rolls up his sleeves and has a stable chair to stand on. You will need to supervise your child at all times if he is standing on a chair, or playing with water. Drying up is another popular and useful activity – give your child lots of unbreakable things to dry, and praise him for his ability and help.

In addition to baking, the most traditional introduction to cooking, children enjoy other areas of food preparation, too.

* Given a selection of salad ingredients, your child can arrange a delicious salad, using his creativity, with your guidance, as to what combinations might work. You will need to help small children with cutting vegetables (or prepare them ahead), but even the smallest child can help to wash lettuce and add the ingredients to the bowl.
* A fruit salad is a popular and simple dish to prepare. Once you have shown your child how to treat each fruit, he can take on this task by himself. If he is not old enough to use a knife, he can still hull strawberries, peel and divide satsumas, and pull grapes from the stalk. Once peeled, bananas and kiwi fruit are very soft, so these are good fruit to practise cutting with a table knife.
* Teach older children (of ten and over) how to prepare useful components of meals or even whole dishes, such as tomato sauce or omelette, so that this can become their regular 'signature dish', whenever it is required, They will grow in confidence as they carry out these valued jobs.

Tasks for small children

If you think about the tasks involved in your food preparation, there will always be some small way you can include your child. You will not want your child near a hot oven, but he can be happily occupied in little jobs which will keep him away from dangerous situations, such as:

* getting the onions out of the vegetable rack
* finding the tin of tomatoes in the cupboard
* getting the cucumber out of the fridge
* putting paper cases into the tray for fairy cakes
* gently brushing the tops of the uncooked scones or mince pies with milk using a pastry brush

Cooking with older children

Older, school-age children can be trusted to help chop ingredients. Start with mushrooms; they are soft and can be cut easily using an ordinary table knife. Courgettes are also soft to cut. Explain to your child that knives can be dangerous and must be treated very carefully. Tell him that now he is older you think he is very sensible and can be trusted to use the knife properly to help cut the vegetables. Supervise your child at all times, showing him how to hold the vegetable and the knife. If you have a suitable child friendly peeler and demonstrate how to use it, your child will also enjoy peeling washed carrots and potatoes.

As children get older, they love to experiment in the kitchen, adding different flavours and ingredients to cakes, cookies and bread dough – and seeing which ones give the tastiest results. Of course, you will still need to supervise this, but give children as much freedom as possible, only interfering if they want to add something completely inappropriate.

Lessons in the kitchen

There is no end to the knowledge that you can share with your child, and the lessons that can be learned in the kitchen.

* As you cook, talk to your child about what you are doing, such as explaining that we have to peel the onions as we don't eat the skin, and that potatoes need to be cooked before we can eat them.
* Give your child a piece of raw carrot as you prepare them, and then show him how it changes and becomes soft once it is cooked.
* Even making a cake provides an exciting lesson in how the unpalatable raw ingredients are mixed together and cooked to produce something tasty to eat.
* Using tools, such as wooden spoons, whisks and peelers is a good way to develop manual skills.
* Weighing scales provide great opportunities for children to learn about numbers and weights.

Cooking gadgets

Children love machines, and even the most reluctant child can often be encouraged into the kitchen to watch food whizzing round in food processors, liquidisers, juicers and smoothie-makers. You can explain what you are making and what will happen next—whether the food will go in the oven and be made into a cake, become a purée for the baby, or just be poured into a glass and drunk. If you have a rotary whisk, this is great fun for a child, who can turn the handle and watch as the egg mixture is whisked, before it is poured into a pan and made into omelette or scrambled eggs. When using machinery with children, do take care, and never leave your child alone with an electric appliance.

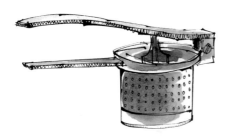

Stress-free baking

You can spend a happy time together baking with your children, but there are a few things worth remembering in order to make the activity as stress-free as possible.

* If you have a baby, plan this activity for a time when the baby is napping, so that you can give your older child your undivided attention.
* Prepare the area where you will be working with your child. Make sure the table or work surface is clean and at the right height for your child.
* Prepare your child. Cover his clothes with an apron, roll up his sleeves, tie back long hair and wash his hands.
* Once you have made and rolled out the dough, your child can press down and cut out shapes using cookie cutters, or make little pastry cups for mini-quiches.
* Remember that, for your child, the pleasure is in the creation, so don't worry if the shapes are not as perfect as you would like.
* Allow your child to get completely involved and to do as much of the task himself as possible. This will give him an enormous feeling of satisfaction.
* Give your child his own piece of dough and a small rolling pin, and let him practise rolling out the dough.
* Don't forget to use flour so that the dough doesn't stick to the board.
* Show your child how to roll gently so that the dough can be lifted off the board.
* Forget about the flour in his hair and on the floor – this can all be cleaned up later.
* Remember, your child will love eating whatever he has made.

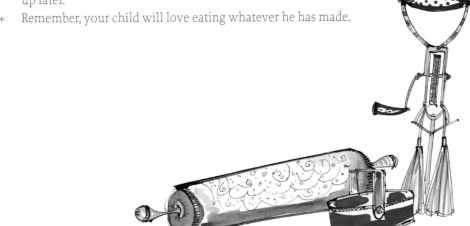

Safety in the kitchen

*   Never leave children unattended in the kitchen.
*   Don't allow your child to stand on an unstable object. If he needs to be higher to reach the work surface, make sure he has a stable stool or a small pair of kitchen steps to stand on.
*   When cooking with children try to prepare everything in advance so that you can concentrate on the task you and your child are doing.
*   Don't try to cook with children if you are in a rush, as accidents are far more likely to happen.
*   Never leave a baby to sit and play on the floor in the kitchen while you are cooking.
*   Tidy away all toys that may be on the floor around you, which might cause you to trip.
*   Keep children away from the hot oven or hob.
*   Always turn saucepan handles inwards during cooking, or when they are on a work surface.
*   Keep your child away from the kettle. The steam produced by a boiling kettle will burn.
*   Teach your child that he must treat kitchen equipment with respect.
*   Keep small children away from dangerous kitchen tools such as knives.
*   Tidy away flexes from electrical appliances so that they are out of reach.
*   Always close cabinet doors and drawers as soon as you have finished using them, to avoid risk of knocks and bangs to the head.
*   Don't allow your child to eat raw cake mixture, because of the risk of salmonella poisoning from raw eggs.

Sweet Treats

There is no denying that sweet foods appeal to children – and often to adults, too. A baby's first foods, such as puréed carrot and sweet potato, are often chosen specifically for their natural sweetness, as it is likely that a baby will enjoy them.

There are many naturally sweet foods, such as fresh fruit, dried fruit and some vegetables, which you can offer your child with an easy conscience, as these foods are highly nutritious. However, be aware that they do contain naturally-occurring sugars and remember to clean your child's teeth twice a day.

If your child is still hungry after his main course and you want to offer him something more to eat, then some chopped fresh fruit or a piece of fresh fruit are healthy options for pudding.

Try to encourage a preference for savoury tastes in your child, rather than a sweet tooth. Don't use sweet treats as a reward or a bribe for your child, as he will then develop an unhealthy connection with sweets and good behaviour.

Puddings are lovely treats for celebrations, parties or a family meal at the weekend. You and your child can have fun making the pudding together and it can become a ritual for all the family. Children appreciate certain foods at special times – you might like to introduce the idea of pancakes (see page 215) for Sunday breakfast. Such happy repetition can make children quite contented.

Making fruit purées

When fruit is in season and readily available you can make delicious fruit purées, which can be frozen for later use. Simmer the fruit (chopped and stoned if necessary) until soft in a small amount of water – just enough to prevent the fruit from sticking and burning. Some fruits, such as blackcurrants,

Sweet treats

Healthy options
yoghurt with chopped fruit, fruit purée or no-added-sugar spread
bowl of fruit salad
puréed stewed fruit—try apple stewed with a splash of water and a
pinch of cinnamon, sweetened with a little honey if necessary

Now and again
pancakes – serve with fruit purée for added nutrition
fruit sorbet
homemade ice lollies
fruit fool—add puréed fruit to custard and Greek-style yoghurt
fruit crumble

Special treats
ice cream
chocolate puddings
sponge puddings
meringues

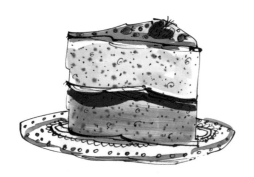

are tart and may benefit from a little sweetener – honey, maple syrup or a little sugar. However, berries are high in vitamin C, so in my opinion the benefit of the fruit's goodness outweighs the disadvantage of needing to add sugar. Once softened, the fruit can be puréed using a hand-held blender or liquidiser and packed in plastic bags or boxes.

Bear in mind that strawberries may not freeze well and are best enjoyed fresh when in season, or to make healthy homemade ice cream (see page 224). Raspberries are extremely delicate and require very little cooking- simmer them for a couple of minutes only until the juices are released, to retain maximum colour and intensity of flavour.

Frozen purées can be used in many ways:
* stir into natural yoghurt for an instant healthy dessert
* mix with custard and yoghurt or cream to make fruit fool
* use to make homemade ice cream
* serve with pancakes (see page 215) or waffles for a tasty breakfast
* offer with a selection of fruit chunks or plain biscuits as a sweet dip for a party
* serve as a sauce alongside cakes and sponge puddings to increase nutritional value – you may wish to add a little liquid if your purée is quite thick
* add to fruit in crumbles – try blackcurrant or apricot purée with apples, and redcurrant purée with plum

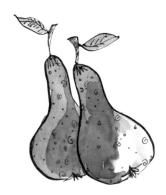

Seasonal fruits to purée

Rhubarb	January to August
Mangoes	imported most of the year; no cooking required when perfectly ripe
Apricots	May to August
Peaches	May to September
Blackcurrants	early July to September
Redcurrants	late June to August
Raspberries	June to October
Loganberries	July to September
Apples	at their best from August to December
Pears	at their best from September to December
Plums	July to October
Damsons	September to November

You can, of course, also enjoy stewed fruit unpuréed. Warm stewed apples in autumn make a delightful dessert, perhaps served with crème fraîche and a dusting of cinnamon. A dish of lightly cooked, jewel-like summer fruits—a combination of any of raspberries, cherries, redcurrants, blackcurrants, blueberries and blackberries—provides a healthy yet sumptuous end to a summer's meal and needs no accompaniment—although Greek yoghurt or good-quality vanilla ice cream would complement it perfectly.

Dried apricots and prunes, available throughout the year, can also be puréed. You will require less purée as the flavour is concentrated in dried fruit.

Chapter 6

Eating Out Made Easy

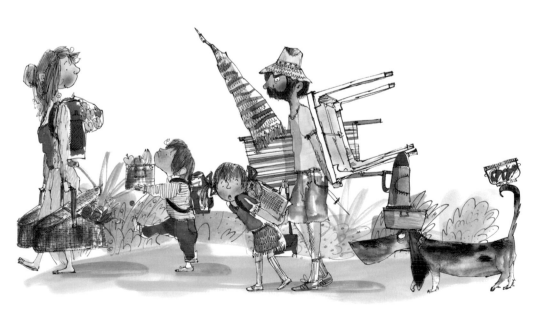

Eating at Restaurants

Although you and your family will be receiving most of your nutrition from home-cooked meals, there may be times when you will want a break from cooking and decide to take the family out for a meal in a café or restaurant.

You want to ensure that your meal out is a relaxed affair for all concerned, so do your homework.

* If you are booking a restaurant in advance, find out whether the restaurant welcomes children, and if they provide highchairs.
* If your choice of café doesn't have highchairs, it is worth investing in a clip-on version, if you intend to eat out regularly. These are also invaluable when you visit friends or family who may not have a highchair.
* Check if there are baby-changing facilities available, if this is something that's important to you.
* Look at the menus of cafés and restaurants before you visit. This saves the inconvenience of having to leave if you discover there is nothing on the menu your child can eat.

For a relaxed visit to a restaurant, ensure that your child is well-rested and is not starving.

Remember to pack everything you will need for your visit. This will include some or all of the following depending on the age of your child:

* a bib
* toys to amuse babies or toddlers; books, crayons and paper for older children
* wet wipes for cleaning sticky fingers and faces
* your child's favourite cup with a lid; even if your child uses an ordinary cup or beaker at home, you may wish to take one with a lid, in case of accidents

As food can take some time to arrive, you may need to amuse little ones with a story book, or some crayons and a notebook. Keep a small bag of café toys in the car or by the front door.

Just because you are away from home doesn't have to mean that your child's diet suffers. So long as you order wisely, you can ensure that they are still getting a balanced meal.

Don't allow your toddler to choose what he wants to eat from the whole menu. You know what is good for him, so give him the choice of two or three options that you have selected. As children get older, they can be allowed more freedom to choose, with your guidance. Restaurant menus often have special children's menus, but don't assume that these will all be designed with nutrition in mind. Beware of the popular chicken nuggets, fish shapes and crunchy dinosaurs. Although these will doubtless appeal to your toddler, they will have very little nutritional value and are highly processed. If children's fish and chips are on the menu, ask the waiter if it is real fish, rather than processed. If you do order this type of meal, you can improve the nutritional content by asking for your child's meal to come with a baked potato rather than chips, and a vegetable, such as peas, alongside the ubiquitous baked beans. You may actually decide that your child will get a more nutritious meal by choosing a half-portion of an adult meal.

If you are out with friends and other children in your group are having chicken nuggets, you might consider offering your child a piece of garlic bread or some fruit juice in place of his usual water with meals, so that he is not disappointed that he is not eating the same as his friends. Alternatively you may decide that it is easier not to make a big scene in the restaurant, and to allow him the nuggets on this occasion. You can always make up for the lack of nutritional value by offering your child fresh fruit on the way home, and a healthier supper. Don't make the nuggets appear irresistible by always denying your child. Besides, you can console yourself that he is much more likely to grow up appreciating good food if he has tried the bad stuff.

A good choice from the children's menu is often a simple pasta dish. If there isn't one available, ask if your child can have a half-portion of an adult version. Popular choices are lasagne and spaghetti Bolognese. Most restaurants will happily serve you some pasta with tomato sauce, or simply some grated cheese, if nothing else appeals to your child. You could enhance this by ordering an extra portion of vegetables from the adult menu.

What to order?

Other menu options that might appeal to you and your child and will provide a suitably balanced meal are:

* Baked potatoes, with either baked beans, cheese or tuna. You may need to ask if a smaller portion is available.
* Soup. Check that this is homemade, as ready-made soups are more likely to contain a large amount of salt and additives.
* Margherita pizza. This basic cheese and tomato pizza can be cut up to provide finger food, which might keep your child busy and content while you enjoy your own meal.
* Cheese omelette. Again, you could order some vegetables to accompany this.
* Fishcakes. Check the ingredients to ensure they don't contain anything unexpected such as chillies.
* Half-portions of adult meals such as risottos, rice and pasta dishes, casseroles and moussakas. Ask the restaurant if it is possible to have a child-sized portion.
* Scrambled eggs on toast.
* Cheese and tomato toasted sandwich.

Water

If you are offering still mineral water to small children while eating out, choose brands that are relatively low in sodium and other minerals. All mineral water is required by law to include the typical mineral analysis on the label, so ask to see a bottle before you order. If the mineral content is high, you may wish to choose tap water instead.

Eating out as a family offers an ideal opportunity for children to try new flavours and unusual foods. You could select something familiar for your child, but order something for yourself that your child has never eaten. Make a show of how delicious your meal is and casually offer some to other members of the family to taste. In this relaxed, unpressurised environment, children may enjoy trying new foods, particularly from someone else's plate, and this may be an easy way of widening the selection of foods they will eat.

The best nutrition

* For the healthiest options, choose dishes that have been grilled, boiled, poached, steamed or stir fried.
* Always ask how something is cooked if you are not sure.
* Ask for dressings to be served separately so you can regulate how much is added.
* Ask for your child's meal to be prepared without salt, if this is possible.
* Ask for vegetables to be served without the addition of butter.
* Don't allow your child to fill up on too much bread or breadsticks before the meal.
* Choose tomato or vegetable-based sauces for pasta, rather than cream or cheese-based ones.
* For a healthy dessert go for fruit sorbets or fruit salad.
* Include a glass of pure fruit juice with your child's meal, as this can count as one of their five-a-day portions of fruit and vegetables. The vitamin C in it also aids the body's absorption of iron from non-meat foods in the meal.

Table manners

Don't be nervous of visiting restaurants with small children. If you are properly prepared, you will be surprised by how well children can behave. They will learn from and imitate the good behaviour around them. Eating out provides the ideal opportunity to teach children about good table manners – sitting still, not leaving the table, holding a knife and fork correctly, using a napkin, talking quietly, eating with their mouth closed, not talking while eating. These are all things that adults take for granted, but are forms of behaviour that need to be taught, and where better to practise than at a restaurant where you have not had to cook the food, too.

If you have a very young baby, feed him at home before you visit the restaurant if possible. This ensures that one member of the family is less likely to cause a disruption during the meal, and allows you to focus on your older child.

Eating on Journeys

Children react very differently to long journeys by car or train. Some will happily look at picture books, watch the passing scenery and listen to story CDs and nursery rhymes; others are easily bored and frustrated, and dislike the confinement of the car seat.

One thing which all children have in common, however, is the need for food and drinks on these occasions. Mealtimes on the road can be fun, and do help to pass the time, but they require careful planning. It can be all too easy to end up serving endless packets of crisps and brightly-wrapped chocolate bars, if you haven't thought about your child's requirements.

Transport tips

* For a long car or train journey with children, you will need to take plenty of snacks that are nutritious, interesting, easy to eat and, crucially, easy to transport.

* If you and your child are often out and about, it is worth investing in a selection of plastic containers in a range of sizes, in which to pack your food. Make sure that your boxes have reliable, leak-proof lids.

* Children like to have their own individual container of little sandwiches. As well as acting as a crumb collector, this will save you handing out each sandwich across a crowded train carriage, and will limit the opportunity for sandwiches getting stuck under the seats of your car.

Food to go

* Mini-finger-sandwiches are more appealing and manageable for little hands, and your child will probably want to eat little and often on a journey. Choose fillings that will stick the sandwich together, such as peanut butter, hummus, cream cheese or Marmite. Remember that Marmite is high in salt, so only use a tiny amount. Select cream cheese carefully, too, as some varieties are higher in salt than others.

* Dry snacks like rice cakes, breadsticks and oatcakes are always useful. Oatcakes often come in convenient sachets within the box – keep a pack in your bag or car's glove compartment.

* If your child likes salad, it may be easier to serve this in a separate little box, as lettuce, tomato and cucumber are notorious for falling out of sandwiches.

* Decant small amounts of hummus or other savoury dips (see pages 220–1) into tiny pots and take along another tub of crudités to dunk in the dips, such as carrots, celery, red and yellow pepper, cucumber and breadsticks.

* Pots of chopped-up fruit are a welcome, thirst-quenching snack. Give each child a colourful selection of fruit to keep their interest.

* Fresh fruit is nutritious and can while away a little time. Choose easily transportable fruit such as small apples, bananas, grapes and satsumas.

* Flapjacks or mini-muffins individually wrapped in greaseproof paper or tin foil will seem exciting, and provide energy to flagging children.

* If you do take ready-made sweet snacks, choose cereal-type bars. Although these still contain a lot of sugar, the oats (or grains) and fruit in them will provide more energy and nutrition than a chocolate biscuit bar – and make a lot less mess.
* Take some little boxes of raisins or a little of pot of dried fruit to distract bored toddlers and keep up energy levels.

Drinks

* It is important to provide plenty of fluids for long journeys to prevent your child becoming dehydrated.
* You can buy children's drinks bottles with anti-spill sports lids, which can be filled with water or diluted fruit juice.
* Bottles of still water are the best option – again, look for the ones with easy-to-use sports tops to cut down on spillages.
* Individual cartons of healthy fruit juice with a straw make a welcome change, but do avoid carbonated drinks and fruit drinks laden with sugar (or sweetener).

Travel essentials

The more thoroughly you are prepared for all eventualities, the more enjoyable your journey will be.

* A pack of wet wipes or a damp flannel in a zip-lock plastic bag is invaluable for wiping sticky fingers and faces.
* A supply of kitchen towel can be useful for clearing up any spills that are likely to happen.
* A change of clothes, in case of any larger spillages.
* A bag of picture books for children to look at will while away the time.
* A selection of small toys or a drawing book and a packet of crayons is invaluable if you are on a train with a table in front of you.
* A few CDs of stories and songs can provide a useful distraction. It may be worth investing in a child's personal CD player if you are frequent train travellers.

Picnics

One of the best things about the summer is that it provides plenty of opportunities to eat outside and have picnics. Children adore picnics and you can make even the most ordinary meal into an occasion just by serving it on a rug in the garden or the park.

There are two kinds of picnic. There is the kind which you plan, down to the last cherry tomato, as part of a family day out or for a celebration (you may be simply celebrating the fact that the sun has shone for two days in a row). Then there is the more spontaneous affair, where you arrange to meet friends in the park with a rug and some sandwiches. The thing which unites all picnics is that they are fun, relaxed occasions. Children can often be persuaded to try something new when you are in this informal setting. If your child is a fussy eater this is the time to not worry. Picnics are all about taking it easy; enjoy each other's company and make the most of this time with family and friends, when there are no chores to do, or daytime interruptions.

Picnic equipment

You will require different foods depending on your type of picnic, but there are some items which will make your life easier whatever the occasion. Wherever you plan to eat, the basic equipment you will need includes:

* a picnic rug or blanket – preferably two
* a suitable carrier for food – cool boxes are ideal, and insulated back-packs leave your hands free to hold little hands
* frozen ice blocks to keep food cool
* a supply of wet wipes

* tea towels and kitchen towel to wipe up spills
* plastic bags to take home any rubbish
* unbreakable plates, bowls and cups as necessary
* paper napkins

Individual containers of food are popular with children, but if you are feeding several children you might like to take some colourful plastic plates or bowls with you.

Buying your picnic

If you don't want to cook and are lucky enough to be near a delicatessen, specialist shop or local farmers' market, you can take advantage of all they have to offer, selecting a variety of cooked meats, cheeses, pâtés and antipasti. Or, for a trouble-free, spontaneous picnic, stop at your local supermarket and pick up ready-made food from the chiller cabinet. Choose wholesome salads and healthy dips, along with pre-prepared crudités and breadsticks. Don't forget plenty of fresh fruit and bottles of water.

For a special, planned-ahead picnic, whatever you prepare, hand-held food is still ideal, so think of things such as:
* mini-sausages, cooked in honey and grainy mustard
* little quiches
* small slices of cold pizza
* child-size sausage rolls
* samosas
* pieces of cold frittata
* hard-boiled eggs in their shells – fun to unwrap and eat whole or quartered

Sandwich ideas

Sandwiches are universally popular, easy to prepare and transport. Use mini-pittas, small French loaves, soft finger rolls and wraps for variety. These are convenient to hold and better at containing sandwich fillings than conventional slices of bread.

Sandwich filling ideas:
* smoked mackerel pâté and cucumber
* slices of cooked chicken, avocado (mashed with a little lemon juice to prevent discolouration) and lettuce
* ham, mashed avocado (as above) and cherry tomatoes, halved
* sliced turkey and cranberry sauce
* cream cheese and strips of roasted red peppers
* cream cheese and avocado
* mild Cheddar cheese (grated) and thin slices of apple
* hummus, grated carrot and lettuce
* hard-boiled egg (mashed with a little soft butter) and cress
* smooth peanut butter and sliced banana
* cold sausage (halved lengthways) and mild chutney
* sardines mashed with a little tomato ketchup
* tuna and tinned sweetcorn – add a little French dressing to bind and provide extra flavour

---

Top tip

Dips and crudités are perfect picnic fare, and will ensure that your child eats something fresh and healthy. Cut up plenty of carrots, celery, peppers, cucumber and cherry tomatoes for a refreshing snack served with hummus, bean or avocado dip (see pages 220–1).

Just desserts

* Fresh fruit is essential for a picnic. Apples, bananas, plums or a bag of cherries are all easy to transport and eat. Take a small knife (well-wrapped in a napkin) if you want to cut up apple while you are out.
* Cubes of pineapple or small slices of melon and watermelon are a thirst-quenching treat. Ensure that you wash melons thoroughly before slicing, as bacteria can be present on the skin. Remove the seeds and refrigerate melon slices to prevent growth of harmful bacteria.
* In summer, a punnet of washed, hulled strawberries will provide a perfect end to your picnic – with perhaps a tub of Greek yoghurt or natural fromage frais to dip them in.
* For a more substantial sweet treat, take along homemade cookies (see page 231), flapjacks (see page 217) or tiny squares of a dense, moist cake such as carrot or courgette cake (see page 229).
* Remember, whatever the cause for celebration, this is not the time for fragile desserts.

Drinks for picnics

* Take plenty of water, as children dehydrate quickly when active in the open air and sunshine.
* Use plastic bottles of water, two-thirds full, then frozen. These can be used as ice blocks to keep the food cool, and then drunk when the ice has melted.
* Any leftover water will be useful for washing hands.
* Smoothies are fun and nutrient-rich for picnics. Prepare these at home, chill and transport in insulated flasks. See page 104 for suggested fruit combinations.
* For extra energy, make homemade old-fashioned lemonade (see page 232).
* You can take flasks of tea or coffee for adults. Mint tea is particularly refreshing and travels well.

Contented picnicking

Picnics should be great fun but so that everyone enjoys the day to the full, there are certain guidelines you need to follow to ensure that the food you prepare and eat is safe.

* Always wash your hands before handling any food, and always use clean utensils and containers to prepare and hold food.
* Do not prepare food more than 24 hours before your picnic, unless it is to be frozen. Any frozen food must be completely thawed in a fridge. If possible, prepare food on the day of the picnic.
* Store all prepared foods in the fridge and pack them at the last minute.
* Use an insulated cooler along with frozen ice blocks to maintain the temperature of cold food and prevent bacterial growth.
* Store food in a cooler with ice blocks under and between containers.
* If travelling to your picnic by car, transport the food in the passenger area, if possible, as this will be cooler than the boot of the car.
* Once at your picnic site, keep your cooler box in the shade and covered by a blanket to maintain the cold temperature inside.
* Take plenty of wet wipes to clean everyone's hands before the meal.
* Keep any uneaten foods in the cooler during the meal. Do not allow cold food to sit out in the warmth.
* Keep all food covered to prevent insect contamination.
* Throw away any remaining food as it will have been sitting out for longer than is safe.

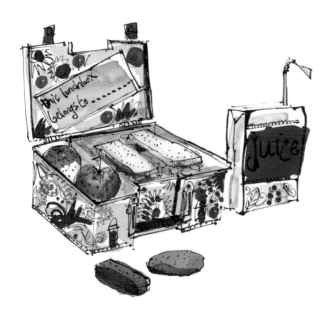

Food that is normally chilled will last for two hours before it should be eaten. This time is reduced to one hour in particularly warm weather. If you cannot keep food cold for long enough, take a picnic of foods which do not require chilling, for example:

* simple sandwiches such as marmite or peanut butter (so long as there are no concerns about allergies)
* breadsticks
* savoury crackers
* fresh unpeeled fruit such as apples, pears, bananas and oranges
* dried fruit
* nuts (if children are old enough and don't have allergies)
* muffins (see page 227) and fruit breads

Accidents can happen

In addition to the food, don't forget to pack a first-aid kit containing insect repellent, antiseptic cream, ointment for burns, bites and nettle stings (the homeopathic Combuduron is an ideal treatment for all of these), arnica cream for bruises, suncream and plasters for blisters and cuts.

Lunchboxes

Once your child starts school, his diet and eating habits take a radical shift. He may be lucky enough to attend a school where they prepare freshly cooked meals using local, well-sourced ingredients, in which case you can relax, knowing that he will receive a nutritious lunch. However, if this isn't the case in your child's school, then it is up to you to provide him with an appetising selection of foods in his lunchbox.

Lunchbox tips

* Invest in some sturdy plastic boxes that are easy for your child to open. You will need a selection of sizes – small ones for items such as chopped fruit and carrot sticks, medium size for rice cakes and oatcakes, and larger boxes for sandwiches or pasta salads. A wide-necked flask is a great idea if your child is allowed to take soup or hot meals in to school.
* Young children starting school can get very hungry and also very tired, so lunchbox foods must be high in energy, easy to eat and instantly recognisable. This is not the time to introduce new flavours or unusual, unfamiliar foods.
* Try to include a variety of foods to ensure that your child receives a balanced and interesting diet. If he doesn't fancy his sandwich, at least he may eat his veggie sticks and dip.
* Write yourself a weekly menu, which removes the frantic last-minute rush to make lunch with whatever is in the fridge. If you know what you are going to provide for your child's lunch you can ensure you add the ingredients to your weekly shopping list.

Suggested lunches for a week

Monday: rice cakes, tuna and sweetcorn wrap, apple, drink

Tuesday: veggie sticks and hummus, cheese roll, grapes, drink

Wednesday: pitta bread filled with cream cheese and avocado, small pot of fruit salad, drink

Thursday: pasta salad, carrot sticks, banana, drink

Friday: wholemeal sandwich with ham and salad, oatcakes, small pot of dried fruit and nuts (if no allergy present), drink

For sandwich filling ideas see page 155.

Making mornings easier

* Weekday mornings are always a rush, especially if you are on your way to work, or there is a baby to feed, so get into the habit of preparing sandwiches and salads the night before and storing them, wrapped and ready in the fridge.

* Make up a bowl of fruit salad and store covered in the fridge for two or three days. You can also serve this for breakfast with yoghurt or cereal.

* You can prepare batches of certain sandwiches (without salad), such as tuna, cheese, ham and cream cheese, and freeze them, taking out what you require in the morning.

* Keep a selection of different breads, ready-sliced, in the freezer. Remove only as much as you need for the day, to provide variety throughout the week, and to preserve freshness. Try granary, multi-grain, bagels, wraps, wholemeal pittas, seeded bread and rolls.

* Batch-cook healthy muffins (see recipes for Courgette Cornmeal Muffins, page 216; Banana Muffins, page 218; Carrot and Pear Honey Muffins, page 227) and store in the freezer, taking them out in the morning. They will have defrosted by lunchtime.

Don't embarrass them

Older children don't like to suffer embarrassment when in the classroom, so pack familiar foods which they are happy to eat in front of their friends.

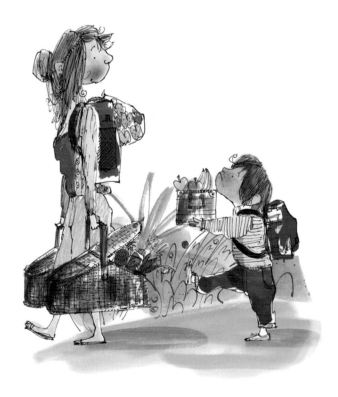

Lunchbox peer pressure

As your child gets older, there may be pressure from contemporaries to include all kinds of packaged and processed foods in his lunchbox. Not only are these expensive but they frequently provide empty calories, filling up small tummies but providing very little nutrition. They may be loaded with additives that could impact on your child's concentration levels. (Additives may also cause disruptive behaviour in some children.) Try talking to other parents and see if you can agree that none of you will provide these foods for your children. If this isn't possible, explain to your child that such foods are for occasional treats and not for everyday meals. If it is becoming a problem for your child, perhaps you could compromise and allow him, say, a small packet of plain crisps or a packaged oat and fruit bar once a week.

Look out for healthier versions of items such as savoury snacks, crisps and flapjacks at health food shops.

School policy

Some schools have a policy against peanut butter in sandwiches, as peanut allergy can be extremely serious, and an allergic child may suffer a reaction from being near someone else's peanut butter sandwiches. There are also some schools that ban all nuts and seeds on their premises. Find out what your school's position is on this.

Ask your child's teacher if there are other foods that aren't allowed in school. You may find that chocolate and crisps are banned, and this makes it easier to explain to your child why he doesn't have them as part of his lunch.

Chapter 7

Recipes

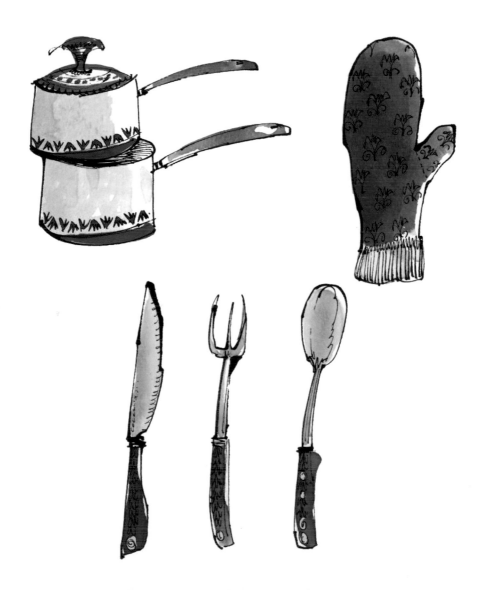

Light Meals

Chickpeas in Tomato Sauce

This store cupboard standby is a great way to introduce children to the earthy softness of chickpeas. Serve on top of millet, quinoa, pasta or couscous, with some grated mild Cheddar cheese or a little Parmesan, or for a more substantial meal, serve alongside grilled chicken or good-quality butcher's sausages. This recipe is suitable for freezing.

SERVES 4
* 1 tbsp olive oil
* 1 onion, finely chopped
* 2 garlic cloves, finely chopped
* 1 large stick celery, chopped
* 400 g can chopped tomatoes
* pinch of chilli flakes or scant ¼ tsp finely minced chilli in oil (optional)
* splash of wine or sherry vinegar (optional)
* 2 x 400 g cans chickpeas, drained and rinsed
* 1 large handful of spinach leaves, spring greens or curly kale, roughly chopped (optional)
* 1 tbsp chopped fresh parsley or coriander

Heat the olive oil in a pan, add the onion and sauté gently for a few minutes until soft, then add the garlic and cook for a further minute or so. Add the celery and sauté for a few more minutes until soft.

Add the tomatoes and chilli, wine or vinegar, if using, and bring to a gentle bubble. Add the chickpeas, and simmer gently for 15 minutes.

Add whatever leafy vegetable you are using and allow it to wilt in the sauce for 5 minutes until tender, then stir in the chopped parsley or coriander.

Sticky Chicken Thighs

The marinade gives the chicken a delicious moistness. This is perfect served with mashed potatoes or rice and your favourite seasonal vegetables. Also great eaten cold for a picnic treat with salads and French bread.

SERVES 4
* 8 chicken thighs, skin on
* 25 g (1 oz) butter
* 2 tbsp Dijon mustard
* 2 tbsp clear honey
* 2 tbsp fresh lemon juice
* 1 tbsp toasted almonds, to garnish (optional)

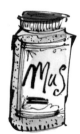

Cut a couple of slashes into the skin of each chicken thigh and place in a non-metallic dish.

Melt the butter in a small pan, stir in the mustard, honey and lemon juice, then leave to cool. When it has cooled down, pour it over the chicken and leave to marinate in the fridge for at least 30 minutes, or preferably overnight.

Pre-heat the oven to 200°C/180°C fan/Gas 6. Place the chicken thighs and the marinade in an ovenproof dish large enough to hold them all in one layer. Cover the dish loosely with foil and bake for about 20 minutes.

Remove the foil and return the chicken to the oven for another 10–15 minutes or until golden brown and the juices run clear when you pierce the thigh with the point of a knife. Just before serving, scatter the almonds over the top of the chicken.

The Best Homemade Lamb Burgers

These burgers are lightened by the addition of some oats and are great for a summer barbecue. Serve in pittas or soft wholemeal rolls with salad and hummus. These can also be made into tasty meatballs to serve with homemade tomato sauce (see pizza recipe on page 182). Smaller meatballs will need slightly less time to cook. The burgers are suitable for freezing.

MAKES 10–12 BURGERS

* 450 g (1 lb) minced lamb
* 75 g (3 oz) rolled oats
* few fresh thyme sprigs, or 1 tsp dried
* 1 tbsp chopped fresh parsley
* 1 onion, finely chopped
* 1 garlic clove, finely chopped
* 1 tbsp olive oil, plus extra for cooking the burgers
* salt and freshly ground black pepper

Place the mince in a bowl and season with a little salt and pepper. Add the oats and herbs.

Fry the onion and garlic in the olive oil for about 5 minutes, until soft but not coloured. Tip into the bowl with the meat and mix together well. Flour your hands to prevent the mixture sticking, then roll the mixture into balls, any size you like (larger for adults and varying in size for the children), then flatten into burger shapes.

To cook, heat a tablespoon of oil in a frying pan and cook gently for 3–4 minutes on each side, until golden brown. Cut one open to check that they are cooked through. Alternatively, grill under a medium heat, turning the burgers until they are cooked through and golden. They can also be barbecued.

Roasted Red Pepper and Feta Frittata

I love to make this for picnics – it tastes even more delicious cold and makes a welcome change from sandwiches. Cut into small pieces, it also makes ideal finger food for toddlers. You can replace the peppers with courgettes, cooked alongside the potatoes, for variety. To reduce the saltiness of feta cheese, soak it in water for an hour before use.

SERVES 6

* 4 tbsp olive oil
* 3 large or 6 medium potatoes, peeled and
  sliced approximately 3 mm (⅛ in) thick
* 1 garlic clove, finely chopped or crushed
* 320 g jar roasted peppers (if in brine, gently
  rinse and dry with kitchen paper)
* 100 g (4 oz) feta cheese, crumbled, or mature Cheddar, grated
* 6 large eggs, beaten
* 75 g (3 oz) rocket or flatleaf parsley, roughly chopped (optional)
* salt and freshly ground black pepper

Pre-heat the oven to 200°C/180°C fan/Gas 6. Line an 18 x 28 cm (7 x 11 in) baking tin with non-stick baking paper.

Heat the oil in a frying pan and fry the potato in batches until golden, then drain on kitchen paper. Add the garlic to the last batch for a few minutes to cook. Do not allow the garlic to burn or it will taste bitter.

Layer half the potatoes in the base of the tin, followed by the drained peppers, then add a layer of rocket or herbs, if using. Top with the remaining potatoes and sprinkle on the feta or Cheddar.

Slightly season the eggs and pour over the vegetables and cheese. Allow to stand for a few minutes to let the egg seep into all the gaps.

Bake for 30–35 minutes until set and golden. Make sure the potatoes are cooked through by testing with a sharp knife. Cut into wedges to serve. Can be eaten hot, warm or cold.

Crunchy-topped Chicken

This tasty chicken dish hides some nutritious nuts and seeds.
Serve with homemade tomato sauce (see pizza recipe on page 182)
and lots of green vegetables. You can make the breadcrumb mixture
when you have a spare few minutes and freeze it, ready to use when
you want a quick meal.

SERVES 4

* 50 g (2 oz) butter
* 2 tbsp clear honey
* 4 tsp grainy mustard
* 1 tsp Worcester sauce
* 4 boneless chicken breasts

TOPPING

* 75 g (3 oz) wholemeal or granary bread,
  made into breadcrumbs in a food processor/liquidiser
* 50 g (2 oz) walnuts, finely chopped in a food
  processor/liquidiser
* 25 g (1 oz) sesame seeds
* 50 g (2 oz) Parmesan cheese, grated
* 1–2 tbsp olive oil

Pre-heat the oven to 180°C/160°C fan/Gas 4.

In a bowl, mix together the breadcrumbs, walnuts, sesame seeds and Parmesan.
Melt the butter in a small pan and add the honey, mustard and Worcester sauce.

Lay the chicken breasts flat in an ovenproof dish and pour over the honey and
mustard mixture. Scatter the breadcrumb mixture over the top and drizzle with
olive oil.

Bake for about 30 minutes or until the topping is golden and crisp and the
chicken is cooked through – the juices should run clear when the chicken is
pierced with a sharp knife.

American Eggy Bread

Perfect for a quick weekend breakfast treat. Without the bacon and maple syrup, this makes a tasty tea for toddlers. Cut into fingers and serve with homemade tomato sauce (see pizza recipe on page 182). For something less sweet, serve with grilled tomatoes and mushrooms.

SERVES 2–3

* 6–8 rashers smoked bacon or pancetta
* 4 slices good rustic bread, crusts removed
* 2 tbsp milk
* 2 eggs, beaten
* sunflower oil, for frying (optional)
* maple syrup, to serve

Fry the bacon or pancetta until very crisp. Remove to a separate plate and keep warm. Also keep the pan warm.

Cut each slice of bread in half. Mix the milk and eggs together in a shallow bowl.

Dip the bread into the eggy mixture and immediately put it into the hot frying pan (there may be enough fat left from the bacon, or use extra sunflower oil).

Fry for a couple of minutes on each side until golden and puffed up and keep warm with the bacon while you cook the remaining bread.

Serve the bread stacked up with bacon on top and drizzle with a little maple syrup.

Variation: Use fruit bread and add a pinch of cinnamon to the egg mixture. Serve with stewed fruit compote or fruit purée (see page 143).

Fruity Chicken

The fruit here adds a rich sweetness to the chicken, making this a hit with all ages. It is delicious served with rice, quinoa, barley, millet or baked potato and seasonal green vegetables. This recipe is suitable for freezing.

SERVES 4–6
* 200 ml (7 fl oz) orange juice
* 1 garlic clove, crushed
* 1 tsp dried oregano
* 75 g (3 oz) dried apricots, chopped
* 75 g (3 oz) dried prunes, chopped
* 50 g (2 oz) *mi-cuit* tomatoes or sun-dried tomatoes in oil, drained
* 4 boneless chicken breasts
* 75 ml (3 fl oz) chicken stock
* 75 ml (3 fl oz) white wine or apple juice
* 1 tbsp brown sugar

Mix together the orange juice, garlic, oregano, apricots, prunes and tomatoes in a non-metallic bowl. Add the chicken, stir to ensure the chicken is coated in the marinade, and leave to marinate in the fridge for as long as possible (1½ hours or overnight if possible).

Pre-heat the oven to 180°C/160°C fan/Gas 4.

Transfer the chicken and marinade ingredients to an ovenproof dish and add the remaining ingredients. Cook, uncovered, for 20–30 minutes. To check if the chicken is cooked, pierce the fattest part of the meat to see if the juices run clear.

Once the chicken is cooked, lift it out of the dish and keep warm while you make the sauce. If you prefer a smooth sauce, transfer the marinade and juices from an ovenproof dish to a liquidiser or food processor and purée it. Or, for a syrupy sauce, boil it in a saucepan rapidly. Return the chicken to the sauce to serve.

Jungle Soup

I call this 'Jungle Soup' as many children like to call broccoli 'trees', and this recipe contains lots of broccoli. It is a perfect way to use up almost any vegetables you may have lurking in the vegetable drawer of your fridge – and who knows what may be lurking in the jungle! Carrots and courgettes make a great substitute for the broccoli. This soup is suitable for freezing.

SERVES 6

* 1 tbsp olive oil
* 2 onions, chopped
* 1 garlic clove, crushed
* 500 g (1 lb 1½ oz) potatoes, chopped
* 1 kg (2½ lb) broccoli, roughly chopped
* 1 litre (1¾ pints) milk
* 1 litre (1¾ pints) chicken or vegetable stock (or you could use a stock cube or vegetable bouillon powder)
* fresh lemon juice, to taste
* crusty bread, to serve

Heat the oil in a large saucepan, add the onions and soften over a gentle heat for 2–3 minutes. Add the garlic and stir for 30 seconds. Add the potatoes and broccoli and stir to coat everything in oil.

When the onions are translucent, add the milk and stock. Simmer the vegetables until they are tender, then purée the soup. Gently reheat the soup if necessary. Add a squeeze of fresh lemon juice to taste and serve with crusty bread.

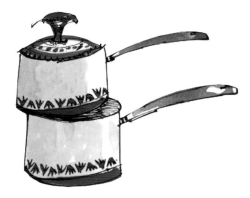

Chicken 'Hiccup'

This dish acquired its delightful name from a young friend who couldn't remember the word for 'Tikka' and came up with this! You can vary the level of spice used in this dish according to your children's taste. Start off mild and you can get progressively hotter as they get older.

SERVES 4–5 ADULTS OR 10 CHILDREN

* 1 kg (2¼ lb) boneless chicken breasts, cut into 2.5 cm (1 in) chunks

MARINADE

* 200 ml (7 fl oz) natural yoghurt
* 1 tsp ground cumin
* 1 tsp ground coriander
* pinch of chilli powder
* 3 garlic cloves, crushed
* 2.5 cm (1 in) piece of fresh root ginger, grated
* juice of half a lemon
* salt, to taste

Combine all the marinade ingredients in a non-metallic dish. Add the chicken and stir to ensure all the chicken is thoroughly coated with the marinade. Leave in the fridge for 1–24 hours, depending on how you will cook it.

Cooking methods:

Stir fry: Add the chicken to a frying pan and stir fry until well cooked. You can add the marinade for more moisture. Serve hot or cold with naan or pitta breads.

Barbecue or grill: If using these methods, try to marinate the chicken for 4–24 hours for the best flavour. Thread the chicken onto skewers and cook, turning regularly, until the chicken is cooked through. Remove from the skewers and serve hot or cold with naans or pitta breads.

Oven cook: Pre-heat the oven to 200°C/180°C fan/Gas 6. Put the chicken in a shallow ovenproof dish. Cover with foil and cook for 30 minutes. Remove the foil and continue cooking for 10–15 minutes until the marinade is brown and the chicken is cooked through. This moister version goes well with basmati rice.

Green Monster Pasta

An excellent, quick tea for hungry children. You can also add a little chopped ham and some quartered cherry tomatoes before serving.

SERVES 2–3 ADULTS OR 4–5 CHILDREN
* 250 g (9 oz) pasta shapes – fusilli works well with this sauce
* 25 g (1 oz) butter
* 1 handful of frozen, chopped spinach or 2 large handfuls of fresh spinach
* 100 g (4 oz) soft cheese with herbs and garlic
* Parmesan cheese, grated, to serve (optional)

Cook the pasta according to the packet instructions.

Melt the butter in a large saucepan and add the spinach. Allow it to wilt (and defrost if frozen) for 1–2 minutes. Add the soft cheese to the pan and stir through the spinach.

Add the cooked, drained pasta to the spinach and stir to combine. Serve with a little grated Parmesan, if required.

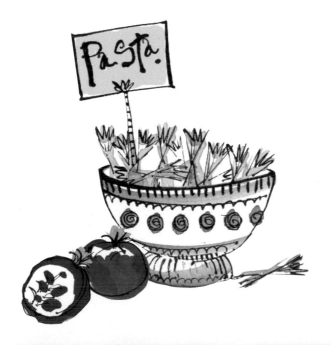

Roasted Vegetables with Couscous

Roasting brings out the natural sweetness in the vegetables, making them more appealing to children. Try also serving this with bulghar wheat, millet or quinoa to increase the variety of grains in your family's diet.

SERVES 4–6

* 3 medium courgettes, halved lengthways and chopped into 2 cm (¾ in) chunks
* 2 peppers, red, yellow or orange, seeded and cut into 2.5 cm (1 in) chunks
* 2 red onions, peeled
* 1 aubergine, halved and quartered lengthways and cut into 2 cm (¾ in) chunks
* 250 g (9 oz) cherry tomatoes
* 2 garlic cloves, finely chopped
* 3–4 tbsp olive oil
* 250 g (9 oz) couscous
* 1 tsp bouillon vegetable powder
* 400 ml (14 fl oz) boiling water
* handful of fresh basil leaves
* Cheddar cheese, grated, to serve (optional)
* salt and freshly ground black pepper

Pre-heat the oven to 210°C/190°C fan/Gas 7.

Carefully slice the peeled onions through the root end in half and then again into the quarters. Cut each quarter in half, making sure the onion stays together at the root.

Place the chopped vegetables in a large roasting tin and toss in the olive oil. Season well.

Roast for 30 minutes, then add whole tomatoes and chopped garlic. Stir everything together, and cook for a further 15 minutes.

Remove the vegetables from oven, and allow to sit while you make the couscous. Place the couscous in a bowl with a splash of olive oil and the bouillon powder.

Pour over the boiling water, stir and cover. Leave to stand for 5 minutes.

Fork through the couscous to break up the grains. Stir the vegetables into the couscous, along with the torn basil leaves. Serve with a little grated Cheddar, if desired.

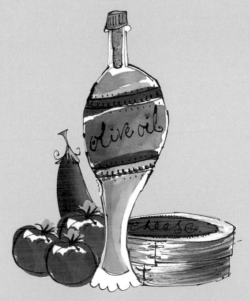

Favourite Fishcakes

Oily fish is a super source of omega-3, so here is an easy and extremely popular recipe for fishcakes using tinned mackerel. Serve with homemade tomato sauce (see pizza recipe on page 182) and plenty of seasonal green vegetables. The fishcakes are suitable for freezing.

MAKES ABOUT 10

* 2 medium–large potatoes, peeled and chopped
* 1–2 tbsp olive oil
* 3–4 spring onions, finely chopped
* 2 x 125 g cans mackerel, drained and mashed
* 1 tbsp chopped fresh parsley
* 5 sun-dried tomatoes in oil, drained and finely chopped
* 50 g (2 oz) fresh wholemeal breadcrumbs

Boil the potatoes in a pan of water until soft, then drain and mash with a fork or potato masher.

Heat one teaspoon of the olive oil in a small pan, add the spring onions and fry until soft. Add to the mashed potato with the mackerel, parsley and sun-dried tomatoes, and combine everything together.

Place the breadcrumbs in a shallow bowl. Take a tablespoonful of the fishy potato mixture and roll into a ball, using well-floured hands to prevent the mixture sticking. Roll in breadcrumbs to coat thoroughly, then press into a flat patty. Repeat with the remaining mixture.

To cook, fry the fishcakes gently in the remaining olive oil for about 3 minutes on each side, until golden brown.

Turkey Burgers

These are a popular and very simple alternative to processed burgers.
Serve in soft wholemeal rolls with salad. The same basic recipe can
also be used to make lamb kofta – replace the turkey with lamb mince,
and instead of making patties, press the meat mixture onto wooden
kebab skewers and grill, turning the skewers, until cooked. The
burgers are suitable for freezing.

MAKES 8–10 BURGERS

* 1 small onion
* 1 tbsp chopped fresh parsley
* 500 g (1 lb 1½ oz) turkey mince
* 1 tbsp olive oil
* salt and freshly ground black pepper
* soft wholemeal rolls and salad, to serve

Blitz the onion in a food processor for a couple of seconds with the parsley and
a little seasoning. Add the turkey mince and pulse just enough to combine the
ingredients. Alternatively, finely chop the onion and parsley and combine with
turkey mince and a little seasoning in a bowl.

Form the mixture into flat patties, approximately 8–10 cm (3–4 in) wide – they
need to be wide as they shrink when cooked.

Fry the patties gently in olive oil for about 3–4 minutes on each side, until cooked
through and golden. Serve one burger each in a wholemeal roll with salad.

Chicken Pitta Pockets

These delicious sandwiches are perfect for a hand-held lunch in the garden, and are equally popular with adults.

MAKES 4

* juice of 1 lime
* 2–3 tbsp olive oil
* 1 tbsp chopped fresh coriander
* 2 skinless chicken breasts, thinly sliced
* 2 tbsp hummus
* 2 tbsp Greek yoghurt
* 1 yellow pepper, thinly sliced
* 4 pitta breads, warmed
* salad leaves, to serve

Mix the lime juice, olive oil and coriander together in a large non-metallic bowl. Add the chicken slices, stir to cover with the marinade, and leave in the fridge for 1–2 hours for the flavours to develop.

Combine the hummus with the Greek yoghurt.

Put the chicken and marinade into a wide, hot pan and cook, stirring, over a high heat until the chicken is cooked through but still tender.

Place the chicken, hummus mixture, yellow pepper and a few salad leaves into the warm, opened pitta pockets.

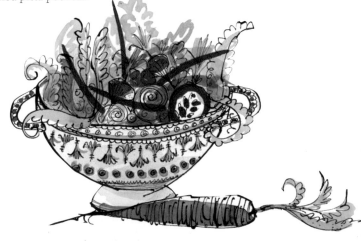

Egg-fried Rice

A great way to use up leftover rice and vegetables, this is equally delicious with brown or white rice. Do not keep cooked rice for more than 2 days in the fridge.

SERVES 4

* 1 tsp olive oil
* 1 tsp sesame oil
* 600 g (1 ¼ lb) of previously cooked rice
* 1 spring onion
* handful of chopped cooked vegetables (e.g. broccoli, courgettes, carrots, peas)
* 50 g (2 oz) chopped ham (optional)
* 2 eggs, beaten
* soy sauce

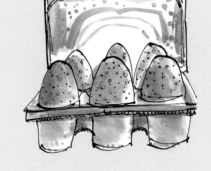

Heat the two oils in a large non-stick pan or wok.

Add the rice and stir fry until piping hot.

Add the vegetables and ham (if using) and stir fry until heated through. Make a well in the middle of the rice, pour in the eggs and scramble until cooked.

Mix the eggs through the rice and add a few dashes of soy sauce to taste.

Serve immediately.

Hearty Bean Soup

This soup, which is almost a stew, can be adapted in so many ways and is a useful store cupboard standby. Try a wintry version adding a leek and using sage and rosemary rather than basil and oregano. You can also add fresh beans or frozen peas near the end. It is delicious served with hunks of crusty bread. This recipe is suitable for freezing.

SERVES 4

* 2 tbsp olive oil
* 1 small onion, finely chopped
* 1 stick of celery, finely chopped
* 2 garlic cloves, finely chopped
* 400 g can cannellini beans, drained
* 400 g can borlotti beans, drained
* 250 ml (8 fl oz) vegetable stock
* 400 g can tomatoes
* 6 fresh basil leaves
* 2 tsp dried oregano
* 100 g (4 oz) pasta tubes
* pesto, to serve (optional)

Heat the oil in a large saucepan over a low heat. Add the onion, celery and garlic and cook over a low heat for 10 minutes until softened but not coloured.

Put a third of the beans into a blender and mix with enough stock to produce a creamy consistency.

Add the remaining stock, 750 ml (1 ½ pints) water, beans (puréed and whole), tomatoes and herbs, bring to the boil and simmer for 10 minutes.

Cook the pasta separately in a pan of boiling water until al dente. Drain and add to the soup. Cook for 5 more minutes or until the pasta is thoroughly cooked, stirring regularly to avoid sticking.

If you wish, add a dollop of pesto to each bowl as you serve.

Chicken Noodle Soup

I call this Japanese-style soup 'Go Fish Soup' as children can fish around for the different ingredients. It works best with a good homemade stock and is extremely versatile. Although I have specified chicken and spinach, tofu and spring greens or prawns and pak choi would work equally well. Look for fresh, seasonal leafy greens. You might need a fork as well as a spoon to eat this!

SERVES 4

* 2 skinless chicken breasts or 4 boneless chicken thighs
* 2 litres (3½ pints) good-quality chicken stock
* 2.5 cm (1 in) piece of fresh root ginger
* 2 garlic cloves
* dash of reduced-salt soy sauce
* juice of half a lemon
* 200 g (7 oz) fine egg noodles
* handful of beansprouts
* couple of handfuls of baby spinach leaves

Place the chicken and stock in a saucepan and bring to the boil. Simmer for about 10 minutes until the chicken is cooked, then lift out with a slotted spoon. Reserve the stock and cut the chicken into thin strips.

Finely chop the garlic and ginger if you think your children will eat it. If not, cut it into larger pieces and remove before serving. Add to the stock and simmer for 10 minutes.

Cook the noodles according to the packet instructions and drain.
Add the shredded chicken to the soup with the soy sauce and lemon juice and cook for 3 minutes. Add the noodles, beansprouts and spinach, stir and serve piping hot.

Pizza

This is a favourite with children – both to make and to eat. Encourage children to try some of the more unusual toppings – they may discover something they like! This tomato sauce is a classic which can be used with all kinds of meals – with pasta or to accompany meat, fish or vegetables, to name but a few. Make a huge batch and freeze for later use.

MAKES 4 SMALL PIZZAS

PIZZA BASE

* 1 quantity bread dough
  (see page 226)

TOMATO SAUCE

* 1 tbsp olive oil
* 2 onions, finely chopped
* 2 garlic cloves, finely chopped
* 400 g can chopped tomatoes
* 350 g jar passata
* 1 tsp dried oregano or
  mixed herbs
* ½ tsp sugar

TOPPING SUGGESTIONS

* grated mozzarella cheese
* chopped ham
* chopped mild pepperoni or salami
* tuna
* anchovies
* pitted halved black olives
* capers
* sliced mushrooms
* sliced red, green and yellow
  peppers
* slices of tomato or halved
  cherry tomatoes
* thinly sliced courgette
* sweetcorn
* chopped fresh herbs, such as
  basil and parsley

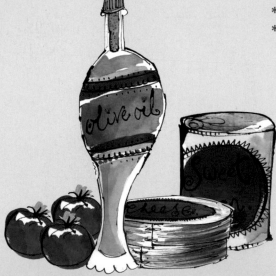

Make a quantity of the bread dough and leave to rise in a warm place until doubled in size.

Meanwhile, make the sauce. Heat the oil in a heavy-based pan and add the onions. Sauté over a medium heat for a few minutes until soft, then add the garlic and cook for another minute. Add the rest of the ingredients, stir well and bring to the boil, then simmer gently, uncovered, for 10–15 minutes until sauce has thickened.

Pre-heat the oven to 200°C/180°C fan/Gas 6. Divide the dough into four and roll out each piece to make flat pizza bases. Place these onto greased baking trays and bake for 5 minutes.

Remove from the oven and cover the bases with a layer of the sauce, followed by your choice of toppings. Sprinkle with dried oregano and return the pizzas to the oven for 10 minutes until the topping is golden and bubbling.

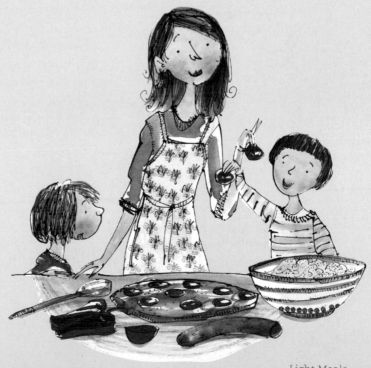

Homemade Pesto

This is so easy to prepare that I recommend you make double quantities and keep a batch of it in the freezer, for an almost-instant and extremely popular meal – and a taste of summer. However, if you are freezing pesto, reserve the Parmesan and add it after defrosting. For variety and a more substantial meal, add any of the following: chopped ham, cooked peas, French beans, sautéed mushrooms, sweetcorn kernels, halved cherry tomatoes. Serve with salad.

SERVES 8–10 HUNGRY CHILDREN, WITH PASTA

* 80 g (3 oz) fresh basil (two good handfuls)
* 50 g (2 oz) Parmesan cheese, finely grated
* 50 g (2 oz) pine nuts
* 150 ml (5 fl oz) olive oil
* 1 small garlic clove, finely chopped (optional)

Wash the basil well and remove the leaves from the tough stalks. Place all the ingredients in a food processor or liquidiser and process everything together until you have a bright green purée. You can add more olive oil if you prefer a runnier consistency.

If you want a milder taste, omit the garlic clove. As an alternative to Parmesan, you can use hard pecorino cheese, which has a more delicate flavour. You can also make this with walnuts or cashews instead of pine nuts, as long as it is not to be served to a child with a nut allergy.

Mini Courgette Rosti Cakes

These make a tasty light tea and are also great served cold in lunchboxes.

MAKES ABOUT 16

* 1 large potato (about 175 g/6 oz), grated
* 1 large courgette (about 175 g/6 oz), grated
* 100 g (4 oz) mature Cheddar cheese, grated
* 2–3 spring onions, finely chopped
* 1 egg
* 2 tbsp plain flour
* 1–2 tbsp olive oil

Mix all the ingredients, except the oil, together in a large bowl.

Heat the oil in a large frying pan over a medium heat.

Drop tablespoonfuls of the mixture into the pan and flatten with the back of the spoon. Cook gently for 3–4 minutes on each side, until golden and cooked through. Serve hot, warm or cold.

Sweetcorn Chowder

This big, nourishing soup is a hit with children of all ages – from teenagers down to toddlers – and their parents. This recipe is suitable for freezing.

SERVES 4

* 1–2 tbsp olive oil
* 1 onion, finely chopped
* 1 green pepper, seeded and diced
* 25 g (1 oz) plain flour
* 1 litre (1¾ pints) vegetable or chicken stock and milk, half and half or to your preference
* 350 g (12 oz) potatoes, cut into 3 cm (1¼ in) chunks
* 250 g (9 oz) frozen, tinned or fresh sweetcorn, drained if necessary
* 100 g (4 oz) Cheddar cheese, grated

Heat the oil in a large saucepan over a low heat. Add the onion and green pepper and cook for about 10 minutes, until softened.

Stir in the flour and cook for 2 minutes, stirring all the time. Add the stock and milk, making sure you scrape any flour off the bottom of the pan and stir or whisk it in thoroughly.

Add the potatoes and cook for 15–20 minutes until potatoes are tender but not collapsing.

Remove the soup from the heat and add the sweetcorn and three quarters of the cheese. Put it back on the heat and bring to a simmer. Serve with the rest of the cheese scattered on top.

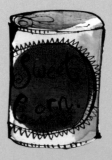

Carrot, Lentil and Sweet Potato Soup

Children love this soup because it's orange and sweet. Parents love it because it's so quick and easy to make and they know their children are getting health-giving carotenoid antioxidants. This recipe is suitable for freezing.

SERVES 4

* 1–2 tbsp olive oil
* 1 onion, finely chopped
* 2 garlic cloves, finely chopped
* 250 g (9 oz) carrots, peeled and roughly chopped
* 250 g (9 oz) sweet potato, peeled and roughly chopped
* ½ tsp ground cumin
* 100 g (4 oz) red lentils
* 1 litre (1¾ pints) vegetable or chicken stock
* fresh lemon juice, to serve

Heat the oil in a large saucepan over a low heat. Add the onion and garlic and cook for 10 minutes until softened but not coloured.

Add the carrots and sweet potato to the pan and cook for 5 minutes. Stir in the cumin and red lentils and briefly cook for 1 minute.

Add the stock, bring to the boil, then simmer, covered, for about 30 minutes until the vegetables are tender and the lentils disintegrated.

Blend and serve with a good squeeze of lemon – children usually like to do this themselves.

Main Meals

Linguine with Tuna and Tomato

Using store cupboard ingredients, this can be put together in about 20 minutes, making it an essential recipe to have up your sleeve. The sauce is suitable for freezing. You can also add 100 g (4 oz) of frozen peas to the sauce 5 minutes before the end of cooking. Further interesting additions include olives, capers and finely chopped courgettes. Serve with salad or crudités.

SERVES 4–6

* 2 tbsp olive oil
* 1 onion, finely chopped
* 1 garlic clove, finely chopped
* 2 x 400 g cans chopped tomatoes
* 1 tsp sugar
* 200 g can tuna, drained
* 500 g (1 lb 1½ oz) linguine or spaghetti
* 1 tbsp chopped fresh parsley
* salt

Heat the olive oil in a large pan and add the onion. Fry gently for 5–10 minutes until softening, then add the garlic and fry for another minute. Add the chopped tomatoes and sugar. Raise the heat and cook for 10 minutes, stirring occasionally. (If you have a very young child or a fussy eater you can liquidise the tomato sauce at this stage to remove traces of the onions.)

Taste the tomato sauce and add the flaked tuna. Keep warm.

While the sauce is simmering, cook the linguine in a large pan of slightly salted boiling water until al dente, then drain.

Add this to the tomato sauce with the chopped parsley and stir well. Traditionally cheese is not served with this dish.

Chicken and Vegetable Stir Fry

You can vary the vegetables in this according to the season. Try broccoli and spinach in winter and courgette batons and finely sliced green beans in summer. Serve with rice, quinoa, bulghar wheat or millet. This is also delicious served with egg noodles, cooked according to the packet instructions and tossed in 1 teaspoon of sesame oil.

SERVES 4

* 1 tbsp sunflower oil
* 1 tbsp sesame oil
* 1 small onion, finely chopped
* 1 garlic clove, crushed
* 4 boneless chicken breasts, sliced into 5 mm (¼ in) thick medallions
* 1 red pepper, seeded and finely sliced
* 200 g (7 oz) mangetout, topped and tailed
* 150 g (5 oz) baby sweetcorn, halved
* 2 tbsp soy sauce
* 2 tbsp chicken stock
* salt and freshly ground black pepper

Heat the oils in a wok or large frying pan. When hot, add the onion and garlic. Stir fry for a couple of minutes, then add the sliced chicken and cook for 8 minutes, until the chicken is just cooked.

Add the red pepper, mangetout and sweetcorn, and continue stirring. Add the soy sauce and stock and simmer for 5 minutes. Check that the chicken is cooked through. Taste and adjust seasoning after serving the children's portions.

Mild Salmon and Coconut Curry

I recommend introducing children to new flavours that all the family enjoys. This gentle, creamy curry couldn't be easier and is a great way to encourage children to try something a bit different. Once they are used to the curry paste, you could add an extra tablespoon for a slightly stronger flavour. Serve with basmati or jasmine rice or some naan bread and your children's favourite vegetables. This recipe is suitable for freezing.

SERVES 4

* 1 tbsp olive oil
* 2 red onions, thinly sliced
* 1 tbsp tikka masala or other mild curry paste (not powder)
* 1 organic salmon fillet, about 600 g (1 lb 4 oz),
  chopped into 2.5 cm (1 in) chunks
* 400 ml can coconut milk
* juice of 1 lime
* large handful of fresh spinach leaves, roughly chopped
* 1 large tbsp chopped fresh coriander

Heat the olive oil in a deep frying pan. Add the onion and cook gently until it begins to soften. Add the curry paste to the pan and heat gently to release the flavours. Add the salmon chunks and cook for 1–2 minutes on each side, just to coat them in the curry paste.

Add the coconut milk and bring to a gentle simmer for 5 minutes. Add the lime juice and taste. Stir in the spinach and allow to wilt. Stir in the coriander just before serving.

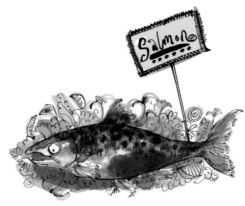

Tagliatelle with Lemon and Courgette Sauce

I love this dish, with its summer vegetables and light lemony sauce. You can replace the broad beans with peas if you prefer. If serving this to toddlers, it may be easier to use pasta shapes such as farfalle, instead of tagliatelle. For a more substantial meal, add 100 g (4 oz) of good-quality cooked ham or smoked salmon before serving.

SERVES 4–6

* 1 tbsp butter
* 1 tbsp olive oil
* 400 g (14 oz) courgettes, sliced in half lengthways and cut into half moons
* 2 garlic cloves, crushed
* 200 ml (7 fl oz) Greek yoghurt
* 200 ml (7 fl oz) crème fraîche
* 125 ml (4 fl oz) single cream
* 150 g (5 oz) broad beans (podded weight)
* grated zest of 1 lemon
* 1 tbsp chopped fresh dill
* 500 g (1 lb 1½ oz) tagliatelle or spaghetti (ideally fresh)
* grated Parmesan cheese, to serve (optional)
* salt and freshly ground black pepper

Melt the butter and oil gently in a large pan, then add the courgettes and garlic and sauté until beginning to soften.

Mix the yoghurt, crème fraîche and cream together and add this to the courgettes, with the broad beans and lemon zest. Simmer the sauce for about 15 minutes, uncovered, until the broad beans are soft and the sauce has reduced and thickened slightly. Add the dill and stir. Taste and add salt and pepper if desired.

Heat a large pan of salted water and bring to the boil. Tip in the pasta and cook until it is al dente. Add the drained pasta to the cream sauce and stir. Taste and add a little more liquid if necessary (either cream or water from the pasta). Serve with grated Parmesan cheese if liked.

Lamb Fillets with Tomato and Mint Couscous

This tasty all-in-one dish is extremely simple and easy-going – it will happily sit for half an hour until you are ready to eat.

SERVES 6
* 2 tbsp olive oil
* 700 g (1½ lb) trimmed lamb fillets, cut into 2.5 cm (1 in) discs
* 1 red pepper, seeded and chopped into 2 cm (¾ in) pieces
* 1 red onion, sliced
* 1 garlic clove, crushed
* 300 g (11 oz) couscous
* 250 g (9 oz) cherry tomatoes
* 600 ml (1 pint) hot chicken stock
* 50 g (2 oz) pitted black olives (optional)
* 175 g (6 oz) freshly cooked peas (frozen are fine)
* 2 tbsp chopped fresh mint

Pre-heat the oven to 200°C/180°C fan/Gas 6.

Heat the oil in a wide, deep flameproof dish with a lid. Brown the meat quickly all over and transfer to a plate. Fry the red pepper and onion for about 5 minutes until they start to soften, adding the garlic for the last minute.

Return the lamb to the pan with any juices from the plate. Scatter the couscous over and nestle the tomatoes amongst it all. Pour over the stock and put the lid on. Place in the oven for 15 minutes.

Remove from the oven, stir and add the olives (if using) and the peas. Return to the oven for a further 5 minutes, then fluff up the couscous and scatter with chopped mint before serving.

Moroccan Lamb and Apricot

The cumin adds a gentle spiciness and the apricots provide a musky sweetness to this popular Middle-Eastern-inspired dish. Serve with rice and a green vegetable such as broccoli or spinach. This recipe is suitable for freezing.

SERVES 4–6

* 2 tbsp olive oil
* 500 g (1 lb 1½ oz) lamb fillet, cubed
* 2 onions, chopped
* 2 carrots, chopped
* 400 g can chopped tomatoes
* 350 g jar passata
* 50 g (2 oz) dried apricots, cut in quarters
* 50 g (2 oz) red lentils, rinsed
* ¼–½ tsp ground cumin
* salt and freshly ground black pepper

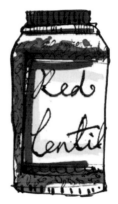

Pre-heat the oven to 130°C/110°C fan/Gas 1.

Heat half the oil in a large, flameproof casserole. Add the lamb in batches and sear, turning, for a minute or so until browned. Remove the lamb to a plate.

Add the remaining oil to the pan, add the onions and cook for about 5 minutes until soft. Return the lamb to the pan, along with the rest of the ingredients and 300 ml (10 fl oz) water. Stir gently and allow the mixture to bubble.

Place a lid on the casserole and cook for 1½ hours. Season to taste with salt and pepper after the children have been served.

Minced Beef Cobbler

This is a traditional recipe in which the 'cobbler' is a topping of savoury scones, which are laid on top of the mince to overlap, like cobblestones. It probably originated as a way of providing a filling meal when there was little more than flour to add to the meat. Children will enjoy helping to make the scones while the mince is cooking. This hearty dish is perfect for providing warmth and energy on cold, winter days. Serve with seasonal green vegetables and any root vegetables, such as carrots, parsnips, leeks, swede, turnip or beetroot. This recipe is suitable for freezing.

SERVES 4–6

* 1 tbsp olive oil
* 1 onion, finely chopped
* 2 celery sticks, finely chopped
* 750 g (1½ lb) lean minced beef
* 1 garlic clove, chopped
* 1 tbsp paprika
* 150 ml (5 fl oz) good-quality beef stock
* 2 tsp tomato purée
* 400 g can chopped tomatoes
* ½ tsp dried oregano or mixed herbs
* 1 tbsp cornflour, mixed to a paste with a little water
* salt and freshly ground black pepper

TOPPING

* 275 g (10 oz) self-raising flour
* 50 g (2 oz) Cheddar cheese, grated
* 1 tsp dried mixed herbs (or 1 tbsp chopped fresh herbs)
* 60 g (2½ oz) butter
* 150 ml (5 fl oz) milk
* beaten egg, to glaze
* 1 tbsp sesame seeds

Heat the oil in a large pan. Add the onion and celery and sauté quickly for 5 minutes, stirring so they don't catch on the base of the pan. Add the beef, garlic and paprika and continue cooking, browning the meat and continually stirring. Stir in the stock, tomato purée, tomatoes and herbs. Simmer gently for 20 minutes.

Add the cornflour paste to the beef mixture, stir and allow to thicken. Taste and adjust the seasoning. Transfer to a shallow ovenproof dish.

Pre-heat the oven to 200°C/180°C fan/Gas 6.

To make the cobbler topping, mix together the flour, cheese and herbs. Rub in the butter with your fingertips until it looks like coarse breadcrumbs. Add the milk slowly, stirring until the mixture forms a soft dough.

Roll the dough out on a floured surface to about 1 cm (½ in) thick, and cut into 5 cm (2 in) rounds using a scone/biscuit cutter. Arrange the scones on top of the mince, brush with the beaten egg and sprinkle with sesame seeds. Bake for 15–20 minutes until the scones are well risen and golden brown.

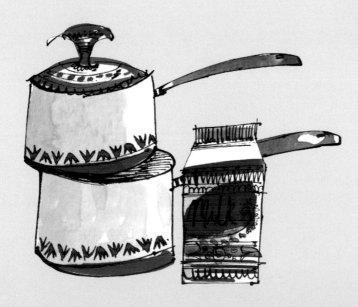

Chicken and Vegetable Bake

This couldn't be easier or more delicious. Use a mixture of whichever root vegetables are in season, such as butternut squash, sweet potato, parsnip, leek and turnip. Serve with a green vegetable or salad.

SERVES 4–6

* 500 g (1 lb 1½ oz) potatoes, peeled and chopped into bite-sized pieces
* 275 g (10 oz) carrots, peeled and chopped into bite-sized pieces
* 2 onions, chopped
* 1 yellow or orange pepper, seeded and chopped into bite-sized pieces
* 2 tbsp olive oil
* 1 heaped tbsp finely chopped fresh herbs – parsley and oregano or thyme
* 1–2 chicken thighs per person, depending on age and appetite.
  (Leave the skin on during cooking to prevent the chicken drying out)

Pre-heat the oven to 180°C/160°C fan/Gas 4.

Arrange the vegetables in a large, shallow ovenproof dish and drizzle with oil. Bake for 20 minutes, then remove from the oven and scatter the herbs over.

Place the chicken thighs on top of the vegetables and return the dish to the oven for about 1 hour or until the juices run clear when the chicken is pierced with a knife and the vegetables are soft. Remove the skin from the chicken before serving.

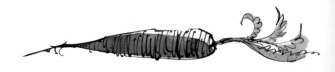

Fish and Prawn Pie with Crunchy Oat Topping

An all-time favourite, this fish pie has a light topping containing healthy oats. Choose any chunky white fish – your fishmonger should be able to recommend something. Children seem to like peas with this, but green beans, broad beans, spinach and broccoli are also good accompaniments. This recipe is suitable for freezing.

SERVES 6

* 1 tbsp olive oil
* 1 onion, finely chopped
* 150 ml (5 fl oz) milk
* 450 g (1 lb) haddock or other white fish
* 25 g (1 oz) butter
* 1 heaped tbsp plain flour
* 1 tbsp tomato purée

* 225 g (8 oz) peeled, raw or cooked king prawns (these can be replaced with more fish if serving to children under the age of two)
* 150 g (5 oz) fresh wholemeal breadcrumbs
* 50 g (2 oz) rolled oats
* 75 g (3 oz) Cheddar cheese, grated

Pre-heat the oven to 180°C/160°C fan/Gas 4.

Heat the oil in a large pan and sauté the onion over a medium heat for 2–3 minutes until soft. Add 150 ml (5 fl oz) water, the milk and the fish. Allow the fish to poach in the gently bubbling liquid for 5 minutes, then remove it with a fish slice or slotted spoon, reserving the liquid.

Melt the butter over a gentle heat in a medium saucepan. Add the flour and stir for a minute. Add a little of the poaching liquid and stir to make a smooth paste. Continue adding liquid, stirring constantly, until you have a smooth sauce. Add some extra milk if you want a thinner sauce. Stir in the tomato purée.

Flake the fish into large chunks, then add to the sauce with the prawns. Place the mixture in a shallow ovenproof dish.

Combine the breadcrumbs, oats and cheese and sprinkle in a thick layer over the fish. Bake for 30 minutes until bubbling and golden.

Turkey and Leek Lasagne

This variation on traditional lasagne is enjoyed by children and is low in fat. A great all-in-one meal, it can be prepared in advance and popped in the oven 40 minutes before eating. It is also a delicious way to use up turkey left over from Christmas. Of course, you can also use chicken. Serve with halved tomatoes, drizzled with olive oil and baked skin-side-down, in an ovenproof dish alongside the lasagne. This recipe is suitable for freezing.

SERVES 4–6

* 1 tbsp olive oil
* 2 medium leeks, washed and finely sliced
* 900 g (2 lb) minced turkey (or chicken), brown or white meat
* 700 g jar of passata
* 1 tbsp tomato purée
* 1 tsp dried oregano or mixed herbs
* 1 tsp sugar
* 2 oz (50 g) butter
* 2 oz (50 g) plain flour
* pinch of dry English mustard
* 600 ml (1 pint) milk
* 100 g (4 oz) mature Cheddar cheese, grated
* 250 g packet easy-cook lasagne sheets
* salt and freshly ground black pepper

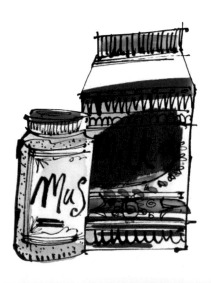

Pre-heat the oven to 200°C/180°C fan/Gas 6.

Heat the oil in a flameproof casserole, add the leeks and sauté until they start to soften. Add the turkey (cooked or raw). Brown slightly and stir, then add the passata, tomato purée and herbs. Season with a pinch of salt, black pepper and the sugar. Cover and place in the oven for 30 minutes.

To make the cheese sauce, melt the butter in a small saucepan and add the flour and the mustard powder. Cook, stirring, for about 1 minute, then gradually add the milk. Whisk to remove any lumps and bring to a gentle boil. Continue stirring until the sauce has thickened, then remove from the heat and stir in the grated cheese.

Remove the turkey from the oven and take the lid off to let it cool a little (do not turn off the oven). Taste and adjust the seasoning.

Spoon one third of the turkey mixture into a gratin dish and cover with a single layer of lasagne sheets. Then top with a third of the cheese sauce. Repeat the whole process twice, finishing with the cheese sauce   you will need about 10 sheets of lasagne altogether. You can scatter the top with a little extra grated cheese if you like.

Return the dish to the oven for 30–40 minutes, until golden brown and bubbling.

Creamy Vegetarian Lasagne

I am a big fan of all-in-one meals, so here iss another one. There is something very satisfying about producing this golden dish, packed with vegetables, knowing it will be enjoyed by all the family. It needs no more than a salad to accompany it. This dish is suitable for freezing.

SERVES 4–6

* 1 tbsp olive oil
* 2 onions, chopped
* 1 garlic clove, chopped
* 2 celery sticks, chopped
* 2 courgettes, quartered
  lengthways and chopped
* 350 g jar passata
* 400 g can chickpeas, drained

* ½ tsp dried mixed herbs
* 25 g (1 oz) butter
* 25 g (1 oz) plain flour
* 450 ml (15 fl oz) milk
* 100 g (4 oz) Cheddar cheese,
  grated, plus extra to sprinkle
* 50 g (2 oz) low-fat soft cheese
* 250 g packet easy-cook
  lasagne sheets

Pre-heat the oven to 200°C/180°C fan/Gas 6.

Heat the oil in a large, heavy-based pan, add the onion and sauté over a low heat until soft. Add the garlic, celery and courgettes and stir. Cover with a lid and cook for a further 5 minutes until the vegetables soften.

Add the passata, chickpeas and herbs and simmer for 5 minutes.

Melt the butter in a medium pan over a low heat. Add the flour and cook for 1 minute. Gradually whisk in the milk, stirring constantly, until the sauce has thickened. Remove the pan from the heat and stir in the Cheddar and soft cheeses.

Place a layer of the vegetable mixture in a shallow, ovenproof dish, followed by a single layer of lasagne sheets and a layer of cheese sauce. Repeat until all vegetables and sauce are finished – you will need about 10 sheets of lasagne altogether. Finish with a layer of cheese sauce and sprinkle a little extra grated cheese over the top.

Bake for about 30 minutes until golden brown and bubbling.

Gently Spiced Monkfish

This is a very mild curry, which children and adults will all enjoy. I like to use monkfish as it keeps its shape when cooked, but you can use any thick white fish or even king prawns. Serve with rice and a leafy green vegetable. This recipe is suitable for freezing.

SERVES 4–6

* 1 tbsp groundnut oil
* 2.5 cm (1 in) piece fresh root ginger, peeled and finely sliced
* 1–2 garlic cloves, crushed
* 1 onion, sliced
* 1 red pepper, seeded and sliced
* 750 g (1½ lb) monkfish, cut into 2 cm (¾ in) chunks
* ½–1 tsp each ground coriander, cumin, turmeric and cinnamon
* 5 cardamom pods, split open by hitting with a rolling
  pin or wooden spoon
* 350 g jar passata
* 120 ml (4 fl oz) Greek yoghurt
* 2 tbsp crème fraîche
* 1 tbsp chopped fresh coriander

Heat the oil in a large pan, add the ginger and garlic and fry over a medium heat for 1 minute until lightly browned. Add the onion and red pepper and allow to soften – this will take about 5 minutes.

Add all the spices and cook, stirring, for 2 minutes. Add the fish and stir to coat with the spice mixture.

Mix the passata with 100 ml (3½ fl oz) water and add this to the fish. Simmer for 10 minutes. Remove the fish to a warm dish.

Add the yoghurt and crème fraîche to the pan and heat gently, stirring. Add the coriander, then return the fish to the sauce to serve. Make sure that you remove the cardamom pods before serving it to children.

Pot-roast Beef

Although this is not a glamorous dish, it is perfect for days when you have been out all afternoon and want to return home to find your meal ready and waiting. If you are lucky enough to have a local butcher, ask him to recommend a suitable joint. You can use any combination of root vegetables in this, including sweet potato, parsnip or turnips. Serve with a green vegetable such as broccoli or spring cabbage.

SERVES 6

* 1 tbsp olive oil
* 1 kg (2¼ lb) beef suitable for pot-roasting, such as middle rib or brisket
* 500 g (1 lb 1½ oz) potatoes, washed, scrubbed or peeled and cut into 4 cm (1½ in) chunks
* 2 red onions, peeled and cut into quarters
* 3 large carrots, scrubbed and cut into 3–4 cm (1¼–1½ in) chunks
* 2 celery sticks, halved lengthways and cut into 3–4 cm (1¼–1½ in) chunks
* 200 g (7 oz) butternut squash, peeled and cut into 3–4 cm (1¼–1½ in) chunks
* a few fresh thyme sprigs or 1 tsp dried thyme
* 400 ml (15 fl oz) hot stock (it is fine to use a stock cube or bouillon powder here)
* 1 tbsp cornflour
* salt and freshly ground black pepper

Pre-heat the oven to 140°C/120°C fan/Gas 1.

Heat the oil in a large flameproof casserole, add the beef and brown on all sides.

Remove the beef from the casserole and add some of the prepared vegetables. Tuck in the thyme sprigs or sprinkle with dried herbs. Sit the beef on the vegetables, and put the rest of the vegetables around it. Season with salt and black pepper.

Pour the stock over the beef. Put the lid on and cook for at least 3 hours. It will be fine if it cooks for longer.

Remove the beef and vegetables to a warm serving dish while you prepare the gravy. Mix the cornflour with a little water to make a smooth paste. Add to the gravy and stir. Check the seasoning and adjust if necessary.

Put the casserole on a medium heat and bring to the boil, stirring, whilst the gravy thickens. Allow the gravy to bubble and reduce a little, before pouring it over the meat and vegetables to serve.

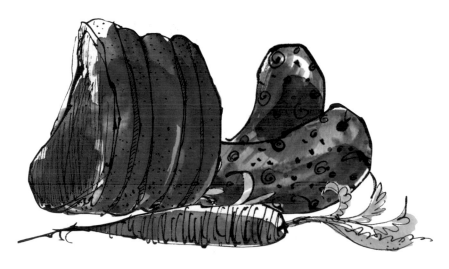

Pot-roast Herby Lamb with Cannellini Beans and Salsa Verde

This dish has all the convenience of a stew. It feeds the whole family and you can prepare it well in advance. The meat is meltingly tender which appeals to young children and the herb-infused lamb subtly introduces new flavours to develop your child's palate. The sharp freshness of salsa verde complements this dish perfectly. Adapt it to your child's tastes; if he finds the garlic or mustard too pungent, leave them out and perhaps add some basil. Serve with seasonal vegetables, and some mashed potato to mop up the meat juices.

SERVES 6–8
* 1 tbsp olive oil
* 2–2.5 kg (4½–5½ lb) shoulder of lamb
* enough fresh sage, rosemary and thyme to thickly cover the bottom of a heavy-based deep pan
* 3 heads of garlic
* a glass of white wine
* 2 × 400 g cans of cannellini beans, drained

SALSA VERDE
* large bunch of flatleaf parsley
* bunch of fresh tarragon
* 20 fresh mint leaves
* 1 garlic clove, crushed
* 100 g (4 oz) capers, drained if necessary
* 2 tbsp red wine vinegar
* 5 tbsp olive oil
* 1 tbsp Dijon mustard

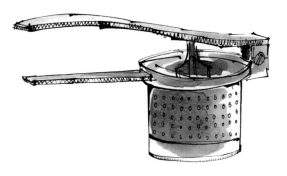

Pre-heat the oven to 200°C/180°C fan/Gas 6. Heat the oil in a large flameproof casserole, add the lamb and brown all over. Don't worry if the lamb only just fits in the dish – it will shrink as it cooks.

Remove the casserole from the heat and lift out the lamb. Line the bottom of the dish with herbs. Cut the heads of garlic in half sideways and place on top, cut-side uppermost.

Put the lamb back in the dish. The layer of herbs and garlic not only infuses the lamb but protects it from cooking too quickly underneath. Cover with a lid and cook for 30 minutes. Turn the heat down to 100°C/80°C fan/Gas ¼ and cook for a further 4 hours (or longer if you wish).

Lift out the lamb. You will find a lot of liquid in the bottom of the pan. This is a combination of meat juices and fat. Use a metal spoon to skim off the fat, which will be sitting on the top. Add the white wine and bring to the boil on the hob. Add the beans and replace the lamb on top. Return to the oven for another hour. To make the salsa, put all the ingredients into a food processor and blend together.

Place the salsa in a small bowl and serve alongside the lamb as required.

Vegetarian Rice

A comforting meal in a bowl. This is a meal in itself, and can also be used as a side dish, served alongside grilled fish or chicken for non-vegetarians.

SERVES 4

* 225 g (8 oz) short grain brown rice
* 1 vegetable stock cube/teaspoon bouillon powder (optional)
* 100 g (4 oz) Puy lentils
* 1 garlic clove, peeled
* 1 bay leaf (optional)
* spring onions, trimmed and cut into 1 cm (½ in) slices
* 1 tbsp vegetable oil
* 225 g (8 oz) fresh spinach, finely chopped
* handful of flatleaf parsley, finely chopped
* 75 g (3 oz) Cheddar cheese, grated

Place the rice in a medium pan, cover with boiling water (adding the stock cube or bouillon powder, if using) and simmer until the rice is tender and the water is absorbed, adding more water if necessary.

Cook the lentils in a small pan of boiling water with the garlic clove and a bay leaf, if available, for 15–20 minutes, until the lentils are soft but still holding their shape.

Meanwhile, sauté the spring onions in the oil in a small frying pan, until soft. Steam the chopped spinach for 1–2 minutes until soft.

When everything is cooked, place the rice and lentils in a large, warmed bowl. Stir in the parsley, spring onions, spinach and grated cheese and mix well. Serve in shallow bowls.

The Best Macaroni Cheese

This is one of my childhood favourites and it is as popular as ever. Serve with lots of green vegetables or salad. This recipe is suitable for freezing.

SERVES 4

* 275 g (10 oz) macaroni, or your child's favourite pasta shape
* 50 g (2 oz) butter
* 1 small onion or a couple of shallots, finely chopped
* 50 g (2 oz) plain flour
* 600 ml (1 pint) milk
* 175 g (6 oz) mature Cheddar cheese, grated
* 1 tsp Dijon mustard
* 2 tomatoes, sliced sideways
* 2 tbsp fresh breadcrumbs
* 2 tbsp grated Parmesan cheese
* sea salt and freshly ground black pepper

Pre-heat the oven to 190°C/170°C fan/Gas 5.

Cook the macaroni in a large pan of boiling, salted water, following the packet instructions.

Melt the butter in a pan, add the onions and cook gently until soft. Stir in the flour and cook very gently, stirring all the time, for about 1 minute. Remove from the heat and slowly add the milk, whisking with a balloon whisk until all the milk is incorporated.

Place back on a gentle heat and bring to a simmer, then stir in the cheese and mustard and season with a pinch of sea salt and black pepper. The sauce should now be smooth and creamy and should coat the back of a spoon.

Off the heat, add the cooked macaroni to the sauce and stir together. Pour into a shallow ovenproof dish and place the tomato slices on top. Mix the breadcrumbs and Parmesan together and sprinkle over the macaroni and tomatoes.

Bake for 20–25 minutes until bubbling and golden brown.

Salad Niçoise

This classic combination of ingredients provides a healthy, well-balanced meal containing omega-3-rich tuna. For children who prefer their food not to be mixed together, place everything in separate bowls on the table and allow them to serve themselves. Encourage them to try a bit of everything.

SERVES 4
* 600 g (1 lb 4 oz) tuna steak, about 1.5 cm (⅝ in) thick
* 500 g (1 lb 1½ oz) new potatoes, scrubbed
* 225 g (8 oz) French beans, topped and tailed
* 225 g (8 oz) cherry tomatoes
* 1 tsp olive oil
* 2 eggs, hard-boiled, peeled and quartered lengthways
* 4 handfuls of salad leaves, washed, dried and torn into bite-sized pieces
* 50 g (2 oz) pitted black olives, halved

MARINADE
* juice of 1 lemon
* 4 tbsp olive oil
* 1 garlic clove, finely chopped or crushed (optional)

DRESSING (OPTIONAL)
* 2 tbsp fresh lemon juice
* 6 tbsp olive oil
* 1 garlic clove, crushed

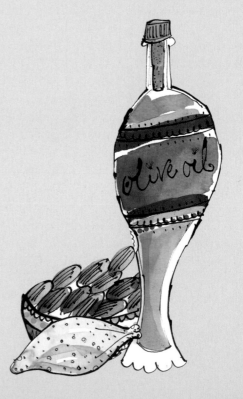

Combine the marinade ingredients together in a screw-top jar. Place the tuna steak in a strong freezer bag and pour over the marinade. Close the bag securely and allow the marinade to coat the tuna. Leave to marinate in the fridge for 30–60 minutes, making sure all the tuna is completely covered by the marinade.

Cut the potatoes in half if they are large, and boil them for 15–20 minutes until tender. Cut the prepared beans in half and fast-boil or steam them for 5 minutes until tender.

Wash the tomatoes and sauté them gently in the olive oil in a heavy-based frying pan for a few minutes until slightly soft. Remove the tomatoes and add the tuna to the frying pan, along with the marinade. Cook the tuna over a medium heat for 2–3 minutes on each side, until slightly brown and cooked through. Check the centre of the tuna with a knife to ensure that it is fully cooked. Do not overcook as the tuna will dry out and become chewy. Cut the tuna into bite-sized pieces.

Combine all the dressing ingredients in screw-top jar. Arrange the salad leaves in a large bowl, and toss with a little of the dressing, if using. Place the potatoes on the salad, followed by the beans, tomatoes, tuna and then the egg quarters. Finish with a sprinkling of olives. Serve with a little additional dressing if desired.

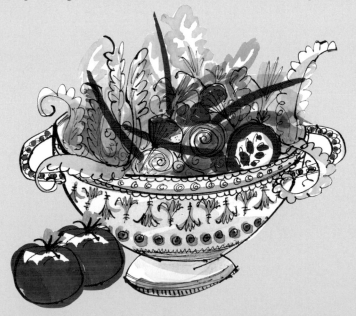

Easy Asian Pork Casserole

This incredibly easy casserole is equally delicious served with either rice and stir fried vegetables or boiled new potatoes and steamed vegetables. This recipe is suitable for freezing.

SERVES 4

* 900 g (2 lb) pork fillet, cut into 2.5 cm (1 in) cubes
* 2.5 cm (1 in) piece of fresh root ginger, peeled and finely chopped
* 150 g (5 oz) pitted prunes
* 3 garlic cloves, bruised
* 250 ml (8 fl oz) apple juice
* 2 tbsp soy sauce
* 1 tsp sesame oil
* 1 tbsp brown sugar
* 2 tbsp hoisin sauce

Pre-heat the oven to 170°C/150°C fan/Gas 3.

Simply mix all the ingredients together in an ovenproof dish. Cover with a lid and cook for 1½–2 hours until the meat is tender.

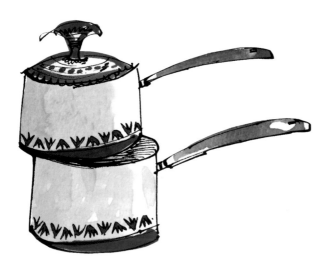

Prawn Risotto

Risottos are one of my all-time favourites and are popular with all ages. Although this one includes prawns, you can use the basic recipe and add different extras such as mushrooms, peas, asparagus and broccoli. Serve with salad or stir through some cooked peas or French beans just before serving.

SERVES 4–6

* 50 g (2 oz) butter
* 1 tbsp olive oil
* 1 onion, finely chopped
* 1 garlic clove, finely chopped
* 350 g (12 oz) arborio rice
* 900 ml (1½ pints) hot chicken stock
* 450 g (1 lb) peeled, cooked king prawns
* 50 g (2 oz) Parmesan cheese, grated
* 1 tbsp pesto sauce (optional)
* basil leaves, to garnish

Heat the butter and oil in a large pan, add the chopped onions and cook gently until soft. Add the garlic and cook for 1 minute.

Add the risotto rice to the pan and stir well to coat in the butter and oil. Add one tablespoon of hot stock to the mixture, and stir. As soon as it has been absorbed, add a ladleful more stock, and continue adding the stock in this way and stirring for about 20 minutes. You want the rice to retain some 'bite', but for the risotto to be quite creamy.

As soon as the rice is cooked, remove from the heat and stir in the prawns and Parmesan (the heat of the rice will heat the prawns in about 5 minutes). Stir in the pesto (if using) and the basil leaves just before serving.

For a vegetarian risotto, replace the prawns with the same quantity of pumpkin or butternut squash. Cut the squash into 1 cm (½ in) cubes and oven-roasted at 200°C/180°C fan/Gas 6 for 20 minutes, until golden and tender. Stir in the Parmesan before serving.

Baked Barley Risotto

Barley is a tasty alternative to rice, and this dish is extremely easy to make. This is delicious on its own, but is also good served alongside grilled chicken, lamb chops or good-quality butcher's sausages.

SERVES 4–6

* 2 tbsp olive oil
* 2 medium leeks, finely sliced
* 1 red pepper, seeded and sliced into 3 cm (1¼ in) batons
* 2 medium courgettes, quartered lengthways and chopped into 1 cm (½ in) chunks
* 200 g (7 oz) pearl barley, soaked in water overnight and drained
* 600 ml (1 pint) vegetable or chicken stock
* 1 tbsp chopped fresh parsley (optional)
* grated Parmesan cheese, to serve (optional)

Pre-heat the oven to 160°C/140°C fan/Gas 3.

Heat the oil in a large flameproof pan, add the leeks, pepper and courgettes and sauté until soft.

Add the barley and the stock to the vegetables and stir. Cover the pan with a lid or tightly-fitting foil and bake in the oven for about 40 minutes, until the liquid is absorbed and the barley is cooked.

Stir the parsley through the risotto, if using, and serve with a little grated cheese if desired.

Baked Fish with Quinoa and Roasted Tomatoes

This is a lovely light and summery dish. I like to stir the tomatoes through the quinoa, but they can just as easily be served alongside.

SERVES 4

* 2 thick fillets of white fish, about 450 g (1 lb)
* 1 small red onion, finely chopped
* 1 tbsp chopped fresh parsley
* juice of 1 lemon
* 4 tbsp olive oil
* 225 g (8 oz) cherry tomatoes
* 100 g (4 oz) quinoa
* 200 ml (7 fl oz) boiling stock (1 tsp bouillon powder mixed with boiling water will be fine)
* 1 tbsp chopped fresh dill
* 2 spring onions, finely chopped
* 100 g (4 oz) broad beans (podded weight) or peas, cooked

Pre-heat the oven to 180°C/160°C fan/Gas 4.

Place the fish in a shallow ovenproof dish, and sprinkle the onion and parsley over it. Mix the lemon juice and half the olive oil together and pour over the fish. Cover the dish with foil and bake for 10–15 minutes. Place the cherry tomatoes in a shallow roasting tin or baking tray, drizzle with one tablespoon of the olive oil, and roast alongside the fish.

Meanwhile, prepare the quinoa. Place the quinoa in a medium pan with the stock, cover with a lid and cook until the water is absorbed – about 15 minutes. Alternatively, place the quinoa and stock in a shallow ovenproof dish. Cover with a lid or foil, place in the oven with the fish, for 20 minutes, stirring once during cooking. Leave the quinoa to stand for 5 minutes, then add the dill and the spring onions, the remaining olive oil and the broad beans or peas.

Serve the fish alongside the quinoa with the roasted cherry tomatoes.

Pasta with Salmon and Broccoli

Another of my all-in-one meals, this is a fabulously easy and tasty way to include some omega-3-rich oily fish in your family's diet. If you want to increase the omega-3 content, stir in a tablespoon of finely crushed walnuts before serving (provided there are no nut allergies).

SERVES 4–6
* 1 tbsp olive oil
* 1 large red onion, finely sliced
* 300 g (11 oz) dried pasta
* 450 g (1 lb) broccoli, broken into small florets
* 400 g can wild red salmon, drained
* grated Parmesan cheese, to serve (optional)

Heat the oil in a large frying pan, add the onion and sauté until soft.

Cook the pasta according to the packet instructions.

Steam the broccoli for about 5 minutes, until just tender, then add to the onion in the pan.

Break the salmon into small pieces and add to the broccoli and onion. (There is no need to remove the bones as the canning process softens them and they are a good source of calcium. I have found to my surprise that children actually enjoy being able to eat the bones in this instance!)

Mix the pasta with the salmon and broccoli mixture and serve in wide bowls, with a little grated Parmesan cheese for non-purists (traditionally, in Italy, Parmesan is not served with fish pasta dishes).

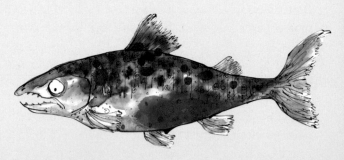

Snacks

Oaty Breakfast Pancakes

These are the small, thicker style of pancakes, perfect for a relaxed weekend breakfast. You could also add a handful of raisins to the mixture. They reheat remarkably well in a toaster, so you can freeze any uneaten pancakes for later use. Do try them using the brazil nuts (if you have no nut allergies in the family) – children who don't like nuts won't even notice the extra ingredient. Serve American-style with maple syrup, or spread with a little butter and pure fruit spread or honey.

MAKES ABOUT 20

* 100 g (4 oz) rolled oats
* 300 ml (10 fl oz) milk
* 200 g (7 oz) wholemeal spelt flour
* 1 tbsp baking powder
* 50 g (2 oz) brazil nuts, finely ground (optional)
* 200 ml (7 fl oz) natural yoghurt
* 1 egg, beaten
* 2 tbsp sunflower oil
* 1 tbsp olive oil

Soak the oats in the milk for 30 minutes before you make the pancakes.

Mix the oats and milk with the flour, baking powder, ground nuts, yoghurt, egg and sunflower oil in a large bowl, to give a smooth, dropping consistency.

Heat the olive oil in a heavy-based frying pan. Using a piece of kitchen paper, wipe the excess oil from the warm pan (don't throw the paper away).

Drop tablespoonfuls of the pancake mixture into the pan, well spaced – you will probably fit about three in the pan at a time, depending on the size of your pan.

Cook the pancakes over a medium heat for 1–2 minutes, until the top starts to bubble. Turn the pancakes over and cook on the other side for 1 minute.

Smear the oily kitchen paper around the pan, to prevent the next batch of pancakes sticking. Repeat this process between each batch of pancakes. Keep the pancakes warm until you have a plateful ready to serve.

Courgette Cornmeal Muffins

These are delicious split and buttered whilst still warm and served with soup. They are also a good savoury snack for hungry toddlers and school children. The muffins are suitable for freezing.

MAKES ABOUT 18

* 150 g (5 oz) cornmeal (polenta)
* 150 g (5 oz) wholemeal spelt flour (ordinary plain flour works well too)
* 1 tsp bicarbonate of soda
* pinch of salt
* 100 g (4 oz) mature Cheddar cheese, grated
* 200 g (7 oz) courgette, grated
* 125 g (4½ oz) butter
* 2 eggs, beaten
* 200 ml (7 fl oz) natural yoghurt

Pre-heat the oven to 180°C/160°C fan/Gas 4. Line an 18-hole deep muffin tin with paper cases.

Combine the cornmeal, flour, bicarbonate of soda, salt, cheese and courgettes in a large bowl.

Melt the butter, then pour into a bowl with the eggs and yoghurt and mix. Add the wet to the dry ingredients and stir gently to combine.

Place dessertspoonfuls of the mixture in the paper cases. Bake for 15–20 minutes until golden brown. Allow to cool in the tin for a few minutes before eating.

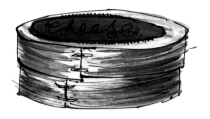

Fruity Flapjacks

Although flapjacks are sweet, the porridge oats and fruit provide a nutritious energy boost – ideal for after-school hunger pangs.

MAKES 16–20 BARS

* 150 g (5 oz) butter or margarine
* 50 g (2 oz) light muscovado sugar
* 3 tbsp clear honey
* 300 g (11 oz) giant porridge oats
* 100 g (4 oz) dried cranberries
* 75 g (3 oz) sultanas
* 50 g (2 oz) chopped almonds or hazelnuts

Pre-heat the oven to 180°C/160°C fan/Gas 4. Grease a 30 x 20 cm (12 x 8 in) shallow roasting tin.

Put the butter, sugar and honey in a medium pan and heat gently until the butter has melted and the sugar is dissolving.

Turn off the heat and add the oats, fruit and nuts and stir until well mixed. Tip the flapjack mixture into the greased tin and level it out. Bake for 15–20 minutes until golden brown.

Allow to cool in the tin for 10 minutes, then mark into squares with a sharp knife. Leave in the tin to cool completely before removing. Flapjacks can be stored in an airtight tin for 1–2 weeks.

Banana Muffins

These are also delicious with the addition of a handful (about 75 g/ 3 oz) of raisins. You could even add a few chocolate chips for a party treat. Make mini-muffins for toddlers and small children and cook for only 10–15 minutes. The muffins are suitable for freezing.

MAKES 12

* 175 g (6 oz) butter
* 50 g (2 oz) caster sugar
* 225 g (8 oz) self-raising flour
* ½ tsp baking powder
* 3 eggs
* 3 very ripe bananas (the riper they are, the more flavour you get)
* 85 ml (3 fl oz) maple syrup

Pre-heat the oven to 180°C/160°C fan/Gas 4. Line a 12-hole deep muffin tin with paper cases.

Using a food processor, whiz together the butter, sugar, flour, baking powder and eggs until well mixed. Add the broken-up bananas and maple syrup and mix until the bananas have been mashed up and the mixture is smooth.

Alternatively, if you are using the wooden spoon method, cream the butter and sugar together and gradually add the beaten eggs. Fold in the flour and baking powder, followed by the mashed bananas and maple syrup. Mix until well combined.

Divide the mixture between the paper cases and bake for 15–20 minutes until well risen and just firm to the touch. Remove from the oven and once cool enough to handle, remove the muffins from tin and cool on a wire rack.

Rye Sticks

A tasty alternative to breadsticks, and great fun for children to help make. The sticks are suitable for freezing.

MAKES 12–14

* 100 g (4 oz) very soft butter
* 200 g (7 oz) rye flour
* 1–2 tbsp milk

Pre-heat the oven to 180°C/160°C fan/Gas 4. Grease a baking sheet.

Rub the butter into the flour until the mixture resembles breadcrumbs. Add enough milk to form a soft dough. Take walnut-sized pieces of dough and roll into sausage shapes – this is something that even the smallest child can do very easily.

Place on the greased baking sheet and bake for 15–20 minutes, until pale golden brown. Allow the sticks to cool for a few minutes on the baking sheet before transferring them to a wire rack.

Once cool, serve plain or with savoury dips, fruit purée, yoghurt or fromage frais. Store in an airtight container for 1 2 weeks.

Three of the Best Dips

Dips are popular with the whole family. Great with chunks of raw vegetables, breadsticks, rye sticks (see page 219) or oatcakes (see page 222), they are ideal for independent toddlers or as an after-school snack, as well as providing a super nutrient boost for hungry parents.

Red Pepper Hummus

The red pepper provides a sweetness to the hummus, as well as packing in some extra goodness.

MAKES ONE CEREAL-SIZED BOWLFUL

* 1 large red pepper, washed
* a little oil, for greasing
* 400 g can chickpeas, drained and rinsed
* 2 tbsp light tahini paste
* 3 tbsp olive oil
* juice of half a lemon
* 1 small garlic clove, crushed (optional)

Pre-heat the oven to 200°C/180°C fan/Gas 6.

Cut the pepper in half lengthways and place, cut side down, on a greased baking tray. Roast for 20 minutes, until it begins to look charred and wrinkled. Remove from the oven and place the pepper in a paper bag for 10 minutes – as the pepper cools, the skin will loosen and become easier to remove. Remove the skin and roughly chop the pepper.

Place the rest of the ingredients, along with the chopped pepper and 1 tablespoon of water, in a food processor or liquidiser and process until you have a smooth consistency. Add a little more water if you prefer a runnier dip.

Store in an airtight container in the fridge and use within 3 days.

Gina's Guacamole

The coriander adds an extra dimension to this avocado-based dip and is a mild, sweet herb often liked by children. Use as a dip with crudités, stuff into pitta pockets with salad, or spread on rice cakes and crackers.

MAKES ONE CEREAL-SIZED BOWLFUL

* 1 large, very ripe avocado
* 1 tomato, seeded and finely chopped
* ½ small red onion, very finely chopped
* juice of 1 lime
* 1 tbsp finely chopped fresh coriander leaves (optional)

Peel and stone the avocado. Mash the flesh in a bowl with a fork until smooth. Add as much tomato and red onion as you require – red onions aren't as strong as white ones but add with caution nevertheless. Add freshly squeezed lime juice to taste. Stir in the coriander, if using.

Store in an airtight container in the fridge and use within 3 days.

Tomato Bean Dip

This is one of my favourite dips, easily made from store cupboard ingredients. Serve with raw vegetable sticks or spread on oatcakes (see page 222), rice cakes or crackers.

MAKES ONE CEREAL-SIZED BOWLFUL

* 400 g can cannellini beans, drained and rinsed
* 6 large sun-dried tomatoes in oil, drained and chopped
* 2 tbsp oil from the tomatoes or olive oil
* 1–2 tbsp milk

Blitz everything together in a liquidiser or food processor until smooth.

Store in an airtight container in the fridge and use within 3 days.

Oatcakes

These are one of my favourite snacks, as befits my Scottish heritage. Oats are often overlooked, but they are highly nutritious, providing slow-release energy. Try these oatcakes spread with any of my dips (see pages 220–21). This recipe is suitable for freezing.

MAKES 16–20

* 225 g (8 oz) rolled oats, ground to medium oatmeal in liquidiser or food processor
* pinch of bicarbonate of soda
* ¼ tsp salt
* 3 tbsp olive oil
* 3 tbsp boiling water
* flour, for dusting

Pre-heat the oven to 180°C/160°C fan/Gas 4.

Mix the ground oats, bicarbonate of soda and salt in a large bowl. Mix the oil with the water in a jug and add to the oats. Mix to a soft dough, adding more boiling water, if required.

Knead lightly on a floured board, then roll out with a rolling pin to a thickness of about 4 mm (¼ in). Cut into rounds using a cookie cutter, and place on a floured baking sheet. This is quite a dry dough, so you may need to add a little more water towards the end if you have re-rolled the dough more than once.

Bake for 10–15 minutes until crisp and beginning to turn golden. Allow the oatcakes to cool on the baking sheet for a few minutes before transferring to a wire rack.

You can also make oat fingers by squeezing the dough into sausage shapes, as in the Rye Sticks recipe on page 219.

Store in an airtight container for up to two weeks.

Puddings and Baking

Magical Chocolate Pudding

Not one for every day, but a delicious pudding for special occasions. The magic lies in the sauce, which develops under the sponge. This has to be one of the easiest puddings to make, and it can be made even more special by adding a large handful of raspberries to the cake mixture. Serve with thick, cold double cream or Greek yoghurt.

* 100 g (4 oz) butter, softened, plus extra for greasing
* 100 g (4 oz) caster sugar
* 2 eggs
* 1 tsp vanilla extract
* 75 g (3 oz) self-raising flour
* 2 tbsp cocoa powder
* 1–2 tbsp milk
* icing sugar, for dusting

SAUCE
* 2 tbsp cocoa powder
* 100 g (4 oz) soft dark brown sugar
* 600 ml (1 pint) hot water

Pre-heat the oven to 180°C/160°C/Gas 4. Grease a soufflé dish or other shallow ovenproof dish.

Cream the butter and sugar together in a bowl with a wooden spoon or with an electric hand whisk, until pale and creamy. Beat in the eggs, one at a time, and add the vanilla extract.

Gently sift in the flour and cocoa, then add the milk, to form a mixture that gently drops from a spoon. Scrape the sponge mixture into the prepared dish.

To make the sauce, place the cocoa and sugar in a bowl, pour on the hot water and mix. Pour the chocolate water over the sponge mixture.

Bake in the oven for about 35 minutes, checking it after 30 minutes. It is ready if the sponge feels firm and springy to the touch. Dust with icing sugar for a professional-looking finish.

Strawberry Yoghurt Ice Cream

Making your own ice cream allows you to control your child's sugar intake. This rosy-pink ice cream is delicious and full of healthy fruit. Full-fat yoghurt should be used or the consistency will suffer.

SERVES 4

* 450 g (1 lb) strawberries, washed, hulled and dried
* 100 g (4 oz) caster sugar (or less depending on the sweetness of the fruit)
* 250 ml (8 fl oz) Greek yoghurt
* juice of half a lemon

Once the strawberries are dry (water will weaken the flavour), place them with the sugar in a liquidiser or food processor and blend until fairly smooth. Add the lemon juice and Greek yoghurt and blend again.

Freeze according to your means – see note below.

If you are storing the ice cream in your freezer (rather than serving immediately), remember to take it out of the freezer and place it in the fridge 30 minutes before serving. This ice cream will keep for a month in the freezer.

Freezing

It is important to whisk air into ice cream to achieve a creamy texture. An ice cream machine will do this for you, but without it, the 'still freezing' method can be used. Pour the unfrozen mixture into a strong plastic box to a depth of about 4 cm (1½ in) and place in the coldest part of the freezer. After 1½ hours, check the mixture. It should be frozen at the edges with slush in the middle. Beat the mixture together with a fork to break up the crystals and quickly return the box to the freezer. Repeat the process twice more and leave in the freezer for at least 1 hour after the last beating before serving.

Banana Loaf

A perfect cake for picnics or a teatime treat. This makes two loaves – eat one straight away and freeze the second one.

MAKES 2 LOAVES

* 2 large ripe bananas
* 100 g (4 oz) soft light brown sugar
* 125 ml (4 fl oz) sunflower oil
* 2 eggs
* 175 ml (6 fl oz) milk
* 175 g (6 oz) wholemeal self-raising flour
* 100 g (4 oz) rolled oats
* 2 tsp baking powder
* ½ tsp bicarbonate of soda

Pre-heat the oven to 180°C/160°C fan/Gas 4. Grease two 1 kg (2 lb) loaf tins and line with non-stick baking paper.

Mash the bananas in a large mixing bowl, then add the sugar, oil, eggs and milk. Stir in the dry ingredients and combine well. Pour the mixture into the two tins.

Bake for 30–35 minutes, or until golden brown and firm to the touch, and when a skewer inserted into the cake comes out clean. Cool in the tins for 10 minutes, then remove and cool on wire rack.

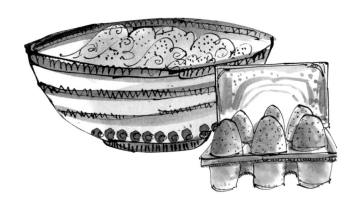

Bread

Do have a go at making your own bread—it's such fun for children to make with you and you will all enjoy eating the results. The bread can be frozen.

MAKES 2 LOAVES, OR 1 LOAF AND 8–10 ROLLS

* 750 g (1½ lb) strong wholemeal or white
  flour or a mixture of both, plus extra for dusting
* ½ tsp salt
* 7 g sachet fast-action yeast
* 425 ml (14½ fl oz) hand-hot water
* 2 tbsp olive oil
* 1 tbsp clear honey

Mix the flour, salt and yeast together in a large bowl. Measure the water into a jug. Stir in the oil and honey. Add the liquid to the flour and stir to form a soft dough. If the mixture is too dry, add more warm water up to a maximum of 175 ml (6 fl oz).

Turn the dough out on to a well-floured board or clean table and knead it for about 5 minutes with the heels of your hands, pushing it away and round in a circular motion, using a firm but light touch. You cannot really spoil this dough, so however you and your child knead it, you will still enjoy a delicious result.

This dough is enough to make two loaves or one loaf and 8–10 rolls. For loaves, divide the dough in two and shape each piece into a smooth oval. These can be placed on a floured baking sheet or in oiled and floured 1 kg (2 lb) loaf tins. To make rolls, divide one half of the dough equally to give 8–10 pieces. Roll each one into a ball and place on a floured baking sheet, with enough space between them to allow for rising. Dust the loaves and rolls with a little extra flour, cover with a clean tea towel and leave to rise in a warm place for about 2 hours until doubled in size.

Pre-heat the oven to 200°C/180°C fan/Gas 6.

Bake the rolls for 10–15 minutes and the loaves for 20–25 minutes. To test if they are done, turn the loaves out of the tin onto a cloth – they should sound hollow when tapped on the base. If they need longer, return them to the oven, but if they are done, leave to cool on a wire rack before eating.

Carrot and Pear Honey Muffins

Children love these unusual muffins – and don't even know they are eating vegetables and fruit! Make mini-muffins for toddler-sized snacks – they will only need to cook for 12–15 minutes. These are also delicious using grated courgette or beetroot in place of the pear. You can also replace the pistachios with cashew or pecan nuts for a change – or leave the nuts out altogether if you are serving these to children with a nut allergy. The muffins are suitable for freezing.

MAKES 12–14 MUFFINS

* 2 tbsp clear honey
* 50 g (2 oz) caster sugar
* 2 large eggs
* 200 ml (7 fl oz) sunflower oil
* 275 g (10 oz) wholemeal self-raising flour
* pinch of salt
* pinch of cinnamon
* 125 g (4½ oz) carrot, grated
* 125 g (4½ oz) pear, grated
* 50 g (2 oz) unsalted, shelled pistachio nuts, finely chopped

Pre-heat the oven to 180°C/160°C fan/Gas 4. Line a deep 12-hole muffin tin with paper cases.

Mix the honey, sugar, eggs and oil together in a bowl.

Combine the flour, salt, cinnamon, carrot, pear and pistachios in a large bowl. Add the oil mixture and stir gently to combine the ingredients. Place dessertspoonfuls into the paper cases.

Bake for 15–20 minutes until golden brown and firm to the touch. Cool the muffins on a wire rack.

Apple and Date Sponge Pudding

A warming autumn pudding – ideal for a weekend family lunch with friends.

SERVES 6

* 500 g (1 lb 1½ oz) eating apples, peeled, cored and sliced
* 100 g (4 oz) dried, stoned dates, halved
* 1 tbsp clear honey
* 125 g (4½ oz) butter, softened, plus extra for greasing
* 100 g (4 oz) soft light brown sugar
* 2 large eggs, beaten
* 1 tsp vanilla extract
* 100 g (4 oz) wholemeal self-raising flour
* 50 g (2 oz) ground almonds
* 2 tbsp milk

Pre-heat the oven to 180°C/160°C fan/Gas 4. Lightly butter a shallow ovenproof dish.

Place the apples and dates in the ovenproof dish, and drizzle with the honey mixed with two tablespoons of water.

Cream the butter and sugar until light and fluffy. Gradually add the eggs and vanilla extract, beating well. Add the flour and ground almonds and fold in gently. Add the milk to give a looser consistency. Spoon the mixture over the apples and dates, and smooth the top.

Bake for 30–35 minutes until golden and firm to the touch. Delicious served with Greek yoghurt, crème fraîche, cream or custard.

Courgette Cake

An unusual, moist and delightfully green loaf cake! A favourite for picnics. This recipe is suitable for freezing.

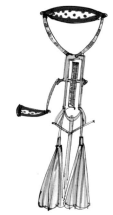

MAKES 2 CAKES

* butter or oil, for greasing
* 3 large eggs
* 225 g (8 oz) sugar
* 2 tsp vanilla extract
* 250 ml (8 fl oz) vegetable oil
* 125 g (4½ oz) grated courgette
* 140 g (4¾ oz) wholemeal flour
* 140 g (4¾ oz) self-raising flour
* ½ tsp baking powder
* ½ tsp salt
* 1 tsp bicarbonate of soda
* 3 tsp ground cinnamon or cardamom

Pre-heat the oven to 180°C/160°C fan/Gas 4. Grease two 1 kg (2 lb) loaf tins and line with non-stick baking paper.

Beat the eggs in a large mixing bowl until light and fluffy. Add the sugar, vanilla extract and oil and blend well. Stir in the courgette. Sift the dry ingredients and add to the egg mixture. Stir until combined. Pour the mixture into the loaf tins.

Bake for 45–50 minutes, until firm to the touch and when a skewer inserted into the cake comes out clean. Cool in the tins for 10 minutes, then remove and cool on a wire rack.

Autumn Apple Cake

I make this cake in a large roasting tin, lined with non-stick baking paper, and freeze half. This is a favourite with children, but is just as popular as a dinner-party dessert, dusted with icing sugar and served warm with cold pouring cream.

MAKES ABOUT 24 LARGE SQUARES
* 3 eggs
* 175 ml (6 fl oz) sunflower oil
* 350 g (12 oz) granulated sugar
* 2 tsp vanilla extract
* 350 g (12 oz) plain flour (or half wholemeal spelt and half white flour)
* 1 tsp bicarbonate of soda
* 2 tsp cinnamon
* ¼ tsp salt
* 2 large cooking apples, peeled and chopped quite small

Pre-heat the oven to 180°C/160°C fan/Gas 4. Grease and line a 25 x 30 cm (10 x 12 in) roasting tin. Beat the eggs and oil together with an electric hand whisk until foamy. Beat in the sugar and continue whisking until the mixture begins to thicken. Add the vanilla extract.

Stir the dry ingredients together in a separate bowl, then gradually add to the egg and sugar mixture, stirring to combine. Stir in the apples.

Pour the mixture into the tin and bake for 25–30 minutes, until golden brown and pulling away from the sides of the tin. Leave to cool in the tin before cutting into slices.

Apricot Cookies

If you want to make these as cut-out decorated cookies for a party,
omit the apricots as they make cutting shapes tricky. This recipe is
suitable for freezing.

MAKES ABOUT 20

* 150 g (5 oz) soft butter, cut into cubes
* 175 g (6 oz) plain white flour or half white and half wholemeal flour
* 50 g (2 oz) ground almonds
* 50 g (2 oz) caster sugar
* 100 g (4 oz) dried apricots, snipped into raisin-sized
  pieces using kitchen scissors

In a large bowl, use your fingertips to rub the butter into the flour and ground
almonds, until the mixture resembles breadcrumbs. Add the sugar and chopped
apricots and continue gently to combine the mixture into a dough. Alternatively,
place all the ingredients in a food processor and process until a soft dough is
formed. Bring the dough together with your hands and knead lightly into a ball.
Place this in a plastic bag in the fridge for 15 minutes.

Pre-heat the oven to 150°C/130°C fan/Gas 2. Lightly grease a large baking sheet.

Take walnut-sized pieces of dough and roll them into balls. Place, well spaced,
onto the baking sheet and flatten with a fork. Bake for about 20 minutes, turning
the sheet round after 10 minutes to ensure even cooking and checking after 15 to
ensure the cookies are not burning. They are best when just pale golden.

Leave to cool and harden on the baking sheet. Store in an airtight container for up
to 2 weeks.

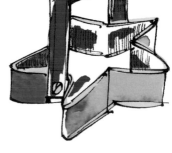

Drinks

Old-fashioned Lemonade

Although there seems to be a lot of sugar in this, it makes about four
bottles of lemonade which is then further diluted to serve. Made at
home, you avoid the additives often found in supermarket squash.

MAKES 4 × 75 ml BOTTLES
* 2 lemons
* 1 orange
* 1.5 kg (3 lb) caster sugar
* 2.25 litres (4 pints) water
* 50 g (2 oz) citric acid (available from pharmacies
  and wine-making suppliers)

First sterilise the bottles you wish to use – old glass bottles with screw-top lids
(such as those used for apple juice or fruit cordial) are perfect.

Pre-heat the oven to 100°C/80°C fan/Gas ¼. Thoroughly wash the bottles and
place them on their sides in the oven for 5 minutes while you make the juice.

Cut away the outer peel of the fruit (discarding the bitter white pith) and blend in
a liquidiser with 300 ml (10 fl oz) of the water for 1 minute.

Pour the lemony water into a large pan with the remaining water and bring
to the boil.

Juice the fruit and add this to the pan along with the sugar and citric acid. Remove
from the heat and stir until the sugar has completely dissolved. Strain into the
hot, sterilised bottles and seal.

To serve, dilute with water (one part juice to six or seven parts water, or to taste).
Store in the fridge and use within one month.

Chapter 8

Meal Planners and Shopping Lists

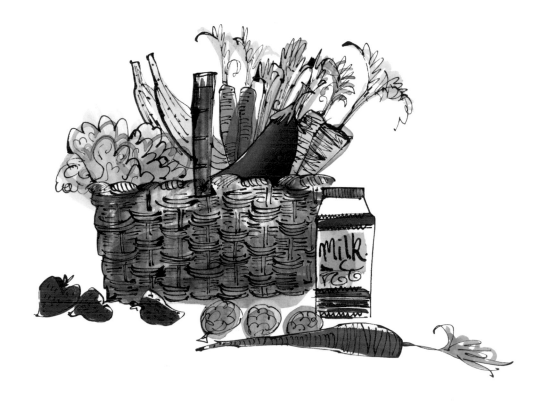

How To Use The Weekly Meal Planners

If you sometimes feel that you are permanently cooking—preparing separate meals for the children and for yourselves—you will benefit from the following plans. These plans are designed so that the same meals can be prepared for both children and adults, even if they are served at different times.

Four-week family meal planner

The following menu plans provide balanced meals for the whole family for four weeks, thereby helping to ease the stress that can arise when one is constantly having to plan what everyone is going to eat throughout the week. Complete with comprehensive shopping lists, you have everything at your fingertips to enable you to provide a range of interesting, tasty meals which will appeal to all the family.

These plans are designed for a routine whereby, during the week, children are served tea at their normal tea-time, while the adults eat later in the evening once the children are in bed. However, weekends are often an ideal time to enjoy meals as a family, which are hugely important and fun for everyone. Most of the main weekend meals can be prepared ahead or involve long, slow cooking—allowing you and your family to get on with weekend activities before enjoying a delicious lunch or dinner together.

Of course, you don't need to follow the entire four-week plan. You might want to start by following the plan for a day or two, perhaps making double and freezing half for later, or you may prefer to use the plan for a week at a time, developing the habit of planning and shopping ahead.

When making baked items like Minced Beef Cobbler, Fish and Prawn Pie with Crunchy Oat Topping, The Best Macaroni Cheese, Baked Barley Risotto, Chicken and Vegetable Bake, and one of the lasagnes, it is a good idea to make a smaller dish for your children and an adult-sized dish so that each one can be baked fresh when needed.

Dishes such as Mild Salmon and Coconut Curry, Chicken and Vegetable Stir Fries, Pasta with Salmon and Broccoli, Roasted Vegetables and Couscous and Gently Spiced Monkfish can be simply reheated for adults in the evening, with fresh rice, pasta or couscous.

Risottos are best eaten soon after their preparation, but can also be reheated. You will need to add more hot stock to loosen the risotto when reheating.

Always ensure that all reheated foods are cooked until they are piping hot and then allowed to cool slightly, if serving to children.

To reduce the amount of your time spent in the kitchen, prepare double quantities of a dish and freeze half for later in the month. On some occasions you will only need to prepare a single quantity and will still have plenty to freeze for later use.

As families are different in both their number and appetite, you may need to alter quantities slightly to suit your requirements. The quantities in these recipes and menu plans should provide plenty for a family of four or five – two adults and two or three children – but only you will know how much your family eats.

Shopping lists

These lists are based on the assumption that you are following the four-week menu plan, and so some ingredients that you buy to use in weeks one and two are also used later in the month, as there will be some left. However, if you just follow week three, for example, you will simply need to check the previous weeks' lists to see if there is an ingredient you need.

If you do intend to follow the complete four-week plan, you should include the quantities in brackets, as these are the additional ingredients needed to enable you to prepare double and freeze half for use later in the four weeks.

Of course, you can choose to buy all the store cupboard ingredients at the beginning of the month, to reduce the amount of shopping trips needed every week. Similarly, you can buy meat and fish in advance and freeze it at home, if space allows. Do remember to check that fish has not previously been frozen, and to ensure that both meat and fish are fully thawed before using.

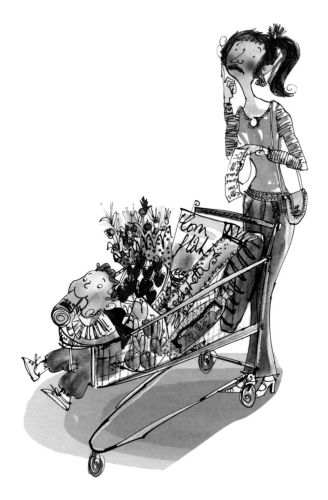

In addition to these lists of ingredients, you will also need a store cupboard containing the following:

olive oil	bouillon powder or stock cubes
sesame oil	Worcester sauce
garlic	paprika
plain flour	dried mixed herbs
self-raising flour	dried oregano
cornflour	dried thyme
rolled oats	chilli flakes
brown sugar	ground coriander
tomato purée	ground cumin
wholegrain Dijon mustard	turmeric
red wine vinegar	cinnamon
soy sauce	cardamon pods

These lists assume that you will be buying milk and also bread (or making it) on a regular basis. You will also need to buy seasonal vegetables and salad to accompany meals, according to availability and your family's requirements.

Week One

Children's Lunch
Children's Tea
Adults' Dinner

Monday

Moroccan Lamb (freeze half for wk 4)
with rice and seasonal vegetables
Sweetcorn Chowder with crusty wholemeal bread
Mild Salmon and Coconut Curry with rice
and seasonal vegetables

Tuesday

Mild Salmon and Coconut Curry (from Monday's Adults' dinner)
with pasta, millet or quinoa and seasonal vegetables
Baked Barley Risotto
Baked Barley Risotto (with Sticky Chicken Thighs–optional)

Wednesday

Chicken and Vegetable Bake with green vegetables
Hearty Bean Soup (freeze half for wk 3)
Chicken and Vegetable Bake with green vegetables

Thursday

Best Macaroni Cheese with seasonal
vegetables or salad
Favourite Fishcakes (make double and
freeze half for wks 2 and 4) with seasonal
vegetables or salad
Best Macaroni Cheese with seasonal
vegetables or salad

Shopping List
Dairy

450 g (1 lb) mature Cheddar cheese
100 g (4 oz) feta cheese
100 g (4 oz) Parmesan cheese
8 eggs

Shopping List
Fresh vegetables

2½ kg (5½ lb) potatoes (+ 500 g/1 lb 1½ oz)
10 onions (+2)
500 g (1 lb 1½ oz) carrots (+ 250 g/9 oz)
1 kg (2 ¼ lb) broccoli
250 g (9 oz) fresh spinach
1 green pepper
1 red pepper
1 yellow or orange pepper
2 red onions
4 medium leeks
2 medium courgettes
head of celery
2 tomatoes
bunch spring onions
fresh parsley, basil and coriander
1 lime
7.5 cm (3 in) fresh ginger (also for wk 2)

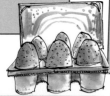

Friday

Fish and Prawn Pie with Crunchy Oat Topping
with seasonal green vegetables
Egg-Fried Rice
Fish and Prawn Pie with Crunchy Oat Topping
with seasonal green vegetables

Saturday

Family Lunch: Turkey and Leek
Lasagne with salad
Jungle Soup with crusty bread
Jungle Soup with crusty bread

Sunday

Family Lunch: Easy Asian Pork Casserole
(make double and freeze half for wk 3) with
mashed potatoes and seasonal vegetables
Roasted Red Pepper and Feta Frittata with salad
Roasted Red Pepper and Feta Frittata with salad

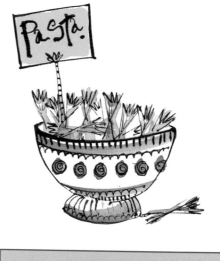

Shopping List
Meat and fish

900 g (2 lb) pork fillet (+ 900 g/2 lb)
500 g (1 lb 1½ oz) lamb fillet (+ 500 g/1 lb 1½ oz)
chicken thighs (1–2 per person)
600 g (1 lb 4 oz) salmon fillet
500 g (1 lb 1½ oz) white fish fillets
200 g (7 oz) king prawns
900 g (2 lb) turkey or chicken mince
50 g (2 oz) cooked ham

Shopping List
Store cupboard ingredients

2 x 400 g cans chopped tomatoes
2 x 700 g jars passata
1 x 250 g can sweetcorn
1 x 400 ml can coconut milk
1 x 400 g can borlotti beans
1 x 400 g can cannellini beans
2 x 125 g cans mackerel in olive oil (+2)
1 x jar sun-dried tomatoes in oil (also for wk 2)
1 x 320 g jar roasted peppers
200 ml (7 fl oz) apple juice
250 g (9 oz) dried apricots (also for wk 2)
250 g (9 oz) dried prunes (also for wk 2)
1 kg (2¼ lb) rice
200 g (7 oz) pearl barley
250 g (9 oz) pkt lasagne sheets
500 g (1 lb 1½ oz) macaroni or other pasta shapes
tikka masala (or other mild) curry paste
small jar pesto sauce
hoisin sauce

Week Two

Children's Lunch
Children's Tea
Adults' Dinner

Monday
Tasty Rice in a Bowl
Best Homemade Lamb Burgers (freeze half for wk 3)
with soft rolls and salad
Vegetarian Rice (with burgers – optional)

Tuesday
Linguine with Tuna Fish and Tomato (make half quantity)
Mini Courgette Rosti Cakes (freeze half for wk 4)
Chickpeas in Tomato Sauce with pasta (freeze half of sauce for wk 4)

Wednesday
Chicken and Vegetable Stir Fry with rice
Carrot, Lentil and Sweet Potato Soup (freeze half for wk 4)
Chicken and Vegetable Stir Fry with rice

Thursday
Creamy Vegetable Lasagne with salad
Favourite Fishcakes (from freezer wk 1)
Creamy Vegetable Lasagne with salad

Shopping List
Dairy

350 g (12 oz) mature Cheddar cheese
100 g (4 oz) soft cheese with herbs and garlic
50 g (2 oz) low-fat cream cheese
4 eggs

Shopping List
Fresh vegetables

700 g (1 lb 11 oz) carrots
250 g (9 oz) sweet potatoes
200 g (7 oz) butternut squash
500 g (1 lb 1½ oz) new potatoes
500 g (1 lb 1½ oz) potatoes + 1 large
6 onions
500 g (1 lb 1½ oz) spinach
bunch spring onions
3 red onions
2 red peppers
500 g (1 lb 1½ oz) cherry tomatoes
250 g (9 oz) French beans
head celery
3 large courgettes
200 g (7 oz) mangetout
150 g (5 oz) baby sweetcorn
large bag baby spinach leaves
small pkt fresh beansprouts
salad leaves
fresh parsley, coriander, mint
2 lemons

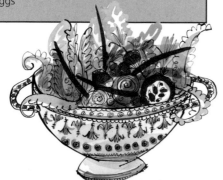

Friday
Minced Beef Cobbler
(freeze half of beef for wk 4)
Salad Niçoise
Salad Niçoise

Saturday
Family Lunch: Lamb Fillets with
Tomato and Mint Couscous
Chicken Noodle Soup
Chicken Noodle Soup

Sunday
Family Lunch: Pot-roast Beef
with seasonal vegetables
Green Monster Pasta
Green Monster Pasta

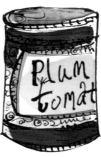

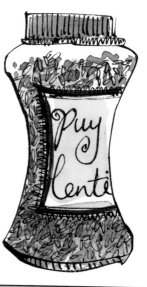

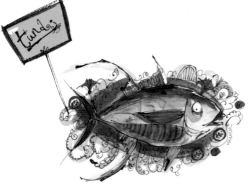

Shopping List
Store cupboard ingredients

3 x 400 g cans chopped tomatoes

1 x 350 g jar passata

3 x 400 g cans chickpeas

1 x 100 g can tuna fish

200 g (7 oz) fine egg noodles

500 g (1 lb 1½ oz) fusilli or other pasta shapes

250 g (9 oz) spaghetti/linguine

250 g (9 oz) brown rice

100 g (4 oz) Puy lentils

300 g (11 oz) couscous

1 x jar pitted back olives (also for wk 4)

100 g (4 oz) sesame seeds (also for wk 3)

75 ml apple juice (+ 75 ml)

soft rolls for lamb burgers

frozen peas

Shopping List
Meat and fish

6 chicken breasts

500 g (1 lb 1½ oz) lamb mince

700 g (1 lb 11 oz) lamb fillet

750 g (1½ lb) lean minced beef

1 kg (2¼ lb) beef for pot-roasting

600 g (1 lb 4 oz) tuna steak

Week Three

Children's Lunch
Children's Tea
Adults' Dinner

Monday
Pasta with Salmon and Broccoli
Best Homemade Lamb Burgers
(from freezer wk 2) with soft rolls and salad
Pasta with Salmon and Broccoli

Tuesday
Easy Asian Pork Casserole (from freezer wk 1)
with mashed potato and seasonal vegetables
Pizza with salad
(Make pizza using half quantity of bread
dough and reserve extra tomato sauce for Friday tea)
Easy Asian Pork Casserole (from freezer wk 1)
with mashed potato and seasonal vegetables

Wednesday
Baked Fish with Quinoa and Roasted Tomatoes
Hearty Bean Soup (from freezer wk 1)
Baked Fish with Quinoa and Roasted Tomatoes

Thursday
Crunchy-topped Chicken (make half quantity)
with seasonal vegetables or salad
Roasted Vegetables and Couscous
Roasted Vegetables and Couscous with salad

Shopping List
Fresh vegetables
baking potatoes for family
350 g (12 oz) potatoes
onions
1 green pepper
2 red, yellow or orange peppers
450 g (1 lb) broccoli
4 red onions
500 g (1l b 1½ oz) cherry tomatoes
100 g (4 oz) broad beans (podded weight)
2 medium courgettes
1 medium aubergine
3 heads garlic
1 lemon
80 g (3 oz) fresh basil leaves
fresh parsley x 2, dill, basil, tarragon, mint,
sage, rosemary, thyme

Shopping List
Dairy
150 g (5 oz) mature Cheddar cheese
150 g (5 oz) Parmesan cheese
2 x 125 g pkts mozzarella cheese
2 eggs

Friday

Prawn Risotto with peas or salad (if serving to under-twos, replace prawns with chopped cooked chicken)

American Eggy Bread with homemade tomato sauce (reserved from Tuesday's pizza)

Prawn Risotto with salad

Saturday

Family Lunch: Shoulder of Lamb with Beans and seasonal vegetables

Sweetcorn Chowder with crusty bread

Sweetcorn Chowder with crusty bread

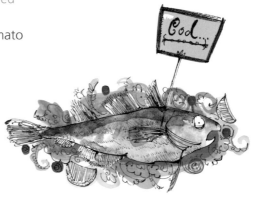

Sunday

Family Lunch: Fruity Chicken (make double and freeze half for wk 4) with baked potatoes and seasonal vegetables

Pasta with Homemade Pesto (freeze half – before adding Parmesan – for wk 4 and later) and salad

Pasta with Homemade Pesto and salad

Shopping List

Store cupboard ingredients

200 ml (7 fl oz) orange juice (+200 ml/7 fl oz)

2 x 400 g cans cannellini beans

1 x 400 g can wild red salmon

1 x 250 g can sweetcorn

1 x 400 g can chopped tomatoes

1 x 700 g jar passata

800 g (1 lb 12 oz) pasta shapes

750 g (1½ lb) strong bread flour

1 pkt fast-action dried yeast (also for wk 4)

250 g (9 oz) couscous

100 g (4 oz) quinoa

350 g (12 oz) risotto (arborio) rice

50 g (2 oz) pine nuts

50 g (2 oz) walnuts

100 g (4 oz) capers

frozen peas

soft rolls for lamb burgers

favourite ingredients for pizza toppings

Shopping List

Meat and fish

6 chicken breasts (+4)

450 g (1 lb) king prawns

450 g (1 lb) white fish fillets

2 kg (4½ lb) shoulder of lamb

Week Four

Children's Lunch
Children's Tea
Adults' Dinner

Monday
Gently Spiced Monkfish with rice and seasonal vegetables
Carrot, Lentil and Sweet Potato Soup (from freezer wk 2)
Gently Spiced Monkfish with rice and seasonal vegetables

Tuesday
Baked Barley Risotto
Mini Courgette Rosti Cakes (from freezer wk 2)
Baked Barley Risotto

Wednesday
Chickpeas in Tomato Sauce with millet (from freezer wk 2)
Favourite Fishcakes (from freezer wk 1)
Moroccan Lamb (from freezer wk 1) with
millet and vegetables or salad

Thursday
Minced Beef Cobbler (from freezer wk 2)
with seasonal vegetables
Pasta with Homemade Pesto (from
freezer wk 3)
Salad Niçoise

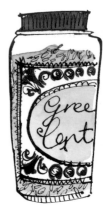

Shopping List
Fresh vegetables
3 onions

2 red onions

3 red peppers

500 g (1 lb 1½ oz) new potatoes

3 large potatoes

2 leeks

2 courgettes

250 g (9 oz) French beans

750 g (1½ lb) cherry tomatoes

100 g (4 oz) broad beans (podded weight)

bunch spring onions

1 lemon

salad leaves

2.5 cm (1 in) fresh ginger

fresh coriander, parsley, dill, mint

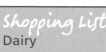

Shopping List
Dairy
125 ml (4½ fl oz) Greek yoghurt

100 g (4 oz) crème fraîche

100 g (4 oz) feta cheese

2 x 125 g pkts mozzarella cheese

8 eggs

Friday

Fruity Chicken (from freezer wk 2) with rice and seasonal vegetables
Salad Niçoise (from Thursday's adult dinner)
Fruity Chicken (from freezer wk 2) with rice and seasonal vegetables

Saturday

Family Lunch: Baked Fish with Quinoa and Roasted Tomatoes with green vegetables
Pizza
Pizza

Sunday

Family Lunch: Lamb Fillets with Tomato and Mint Couscous
Roasted Red Pepper and Feta Frittata with salad
Roasted Red Pepper and Feta Frittata with salad

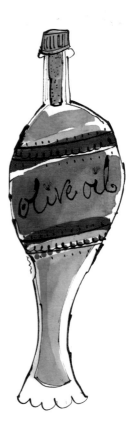

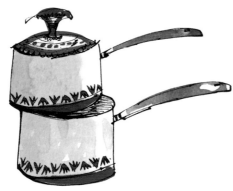

Shopping List
Store cupboard ingredients

1 x 400 g can chopped tomatoes
1 x 700 g jar passata
1 x 320 g jar roasted peppers
500 g (1 lb 1½ oz) pasta
750 g (1 lb 9 oz) strong bread flour
300 g (11 oz) couscous
100 g (4 oz) quinoa
200 g (7 oz) pearl barley
250 g (9 oz) millet
500 g (1 lb 1½ oz) rice
frozen peas

Shopping List
Meat and fish

600 g (1 lb 4 oz) tuna steak
750 g (1½ lb) monkfish
450 g (1 lb) white fish fillets
700 g (1 lb 9 oz) lamb fillet

Chapter 9

Case Studies and Questions and Answers

Case Studies

Refusing Family Meals

Izzy – 21 Months

Kate and David followed the latest guidelines on weaning, and introduced solids to baby Izzy at six months. At this stage she was having five 240 ml (8 oz) bottles of milk, and starting to wake earlier in the morning, so Kate felt confident that Izzy would take to solids really well. But getting Izzy to eat solids was very difficult. It took many months to reduce the milk feeds and get her to eat even a small amount of solids.

By the age of 12 months Izzy would gobble a big breakfast easily, but eat hardly anything at lunch and tea, which were nearly always the same: blended casseroles (lamb couscous, or chicken and veg) and soups (leek and potato, or lentil), followed by fruit purée and yoghurt for dessert. She would not eat vegetables at all unless they were hidden in the puréed casseroles. The only finger foods she would eat were rice cakes, breadsticks or savoury biscuits.

At around 18 months Kate became aware that Izzy's eating habits were very different from those of her friends' children, and play dates and meals at other parents' houses became an embarrassing struggle, as Izzy would refuse the meals that other children were eating.

At 20 months Kate started to try and persuade Izzy to eat a more varied diet. But mealtimes became very stressful. Izzy would spit out any food that contained lumps or vegetables, and eventually started to refuse any type of savoury food, turning her head away when Kate tried to feed her the usual soup or casserole. Kate would end up giving her puréed fruit and yoghurt, along with breadsticks or rice cakes.

By 21 months Izzy was waking up regularly at 5.30am and would not settle back to sleep unless given a beaker of milk. It was at this stage that Kate contacted me. The following food diary showed Izzy's typical daily feeding pattern:

* 5.30am – 180 ml (6 oz) milk
* 7.30am – 180 ml (6 oz) milk, 2 Weetabix or large bowl of cereal plus fruit purée

* 10am – 120 ml (4 oz) vegetable/fruit juice, two savoury biscuits, breadsticks, or rice cakes plus dried fruit
* 12 noon – 2 to 3 tablespoons of puréed savoury meal (refusing lumps), breadsticks or rice cakes, 120 g (4 oz) pot of yoghurt and fruit purée, 30 ml (1 oz) of vegetable/fruit juice
* 3pm – 120 ml (4 oz) milk, dried fruit and 1–2 savoury biscuits
* 5pm – 2 to 3 tablespoons of puréed savoury meal, breadsticks, 120 g (4 oz) pot of yoghurt and fruit purée, 120 ml (4 oz) milk
* 6.30pm – 120 ml (4 oz) milk

I was not convinced that the problem was to do with lumps in food, as Izzy was happy to eat savoury biscuits, etc. However, I did feel that she was eating an excessive amount of carbohydrates in the morning which, together with the milk feeds at 5.30am and 3pm, might be affecting her appetite at lunch and tea.

Because Izzy was genuinely hungry at 5.30am, I suggested that Kate should continue to give her this milk feed, but count it as her breakfast milk and replace the breakfast milk with a drink of well-diluted juice or water for the time being. I then recommended that Kate should adopt the following feeding plan:

* 5.30am – 180 ml (6 oz) milk (gradually reducing this amount once lunch and teatime solids have increased)
* 7.30am – 120 g (4 oz) pot of yoghurt and fruit purée, plus drink of well-diluted juice. Once lunch is well established for at least three or four days, gradually replace yoghurt with breakfast cereal, but no more than one Weetabix or the equivalent. As Izzy sleeps later in the morning, and the 5.30am feed is dropped, then a 120–180 ml (4–6 oz) milk feed should be offered at breakfast.
* 10am – Drink of water and chopped fruit
* 12noon – Savoury lunch with chopped/sliced vegetables, followed by chopped/ sliced fruit if all of savoury food was eaten, plus drink of well-diluted juice or water, but not until Izzy has eaten at least half of her meal. (It is important not to overload the plate. Better to put a small portion of food on the plate and then add to it if required.)
* 3pm – Drink of water and chopped fruit
* 5pm – Baked potato or pasta served with vegetables, or thick vegetable soup served with bread, plus 90–120 ml (3–4 oz) milk
* 6.30pm – 150–180 ml (5–6 oz) milk

As a last resort, if Izzy did not eat well in the evening, she could have cereal so that she was not going to bed on an empty tummy. I also stressed the importance of not cajoling Izzy at mealtimes should she refuse to eat.

Kate was worried that Izzy would be terribly hungry, but I reassured her that Izzy's appetite would very quickly improve once breakfast was changed, the amount of milk she was drinking was reduced, and the carbohydrate snacks were replaced by fruit. She was also concerned that Izzy's milk intake would be too low. But I explained that Izzy would still be drinking 420–480 ml (14–16 oz) of milk a day, which is higher than the minimum recommended amount for a child of Izzy's age (360 ml or 12 oz).

By structuring her food and drink so that the right type of foods were being served at the right time of day, rather than allowing her to fill up on juice and biscuits between meals, I was confident that Izzy would soon move on to eating family-type meals, and increase the actual amounts she ate.

I explained to Kate that it was important to allow a child of Izzy's age some control over how much they wanted to eat, not to force her, and to allow a set time of 20–30 minutes for each meal. If Izzy refused the food or fussed, it should be taken away, and Kate should make no comment whatsoever. Izzy should not be offered any further food until snacktime, and at this stage it should be chopped fruit, not biscuits or breadsticks. Whenever possible, particularly at lunchtime, Kate should try to eat with Izzy.

The first four days of following the plan were difficult for Kate, as Izzy did have several tantrums, and would at times refuse lunch or eat very little. But Kate remained calm and consistent, and stuck with the menu planner I had given her.

Within two weeks, Izzy's eating had improved dramatically. She gradually started to sleep until 6.30am, and Kate was then able to resume a normal breakfast with a drink of milk from a beaker, plus cereal and fruit, replacing the fruit purée with chopped fruit. Kate continued to offer only fruit as a snack, except on play dates when she allowed Izzy a biscuit along with the other children. Izzy would then often eat slightly less at lunchtime, but not so much that Kate was worried about it.

By the end of the third week Izzy was readily eating a wide variety of foods and happily joining in family meals at home and at friends' houses.

Case Studies

Problems With Texture

Harry – 10 Months

At the age of a year, Harry was underweight and only interested in puréed food. He had suffered from reflux since he was eight weeks old, and persuading him to take even the minimum requirement of milk had been a daily challenge for his parents, Tanya and Ivan. Harry had finally started to drink 'enough' milk at eleven months, but his weight gain was still poor and his parents had problems progressing him from puréed food to more textured, grown-up food.

At this point they contacted me. In the first instance I suggested that they focus on Harry's weight gain, which included increasing the amount of solids he ate. Only when this had started to improve would we focus on textured food.

Although Harry had finally started to drink 'enough' milk, this now needed to be reduced to ensure that solids became his main food source. At the age of a year, Harry needed a minimum of 360 ml (12 oz) milk a day, but his daily milk intake was around 630–720 ml (21–24 oz) divided between three feeds. I suggested this should be reduced to around 510 ml (17 oz) a day, and advised his parents to give him 150 ml (5 oz) first thing in the morning and again mid-afternoon, followed by 210 ml (7 oz) in the evening. I also suggested that Ivan and Tanya change their 'hungrier baby' formula, which is more filling, back to first-stage milk.

This advice worked almost immediately. With less milk over the course of a day, Harry ate larger portions of the puréed foods he loved, and I advised Tanya to add fat and calories where possible – butter, cheese, full-fat milk, olive oil, etc. After a month, Tanya and Ivan were thrilled to see that Harry had begun to put on weight.

During this time, Tanya always offered finger foods, and although Harry was happy to take toast, rice cakes and soft biscuits, most other foods were rejected. However, she always made sure she had something new for him to try.

Once Harry had starting putting on weight, Tanya kept offering him his favourite foods but added to different, slightly more textured foods – for example, soft cubes of vegetables/batons, or pasta in a smooth sauce. At first Harry didn't seem to enjoy them. He would more often than not spit the bits out, or reject the food altogether. Tanya kept on trying, but ensured he was also given meals he would eat happily.

At this point I suggested that Tanya start cutting down on Harry's afternoon milk. He didn't seem as hungry for it any more and often only took 30–60 ml (1–2 oz), so she didn't press him to finish it, just making sure that he had water when he needed it.

Unfortunately, it was at this stage that Harry, during a visit to his Granny's, managed to grab the hot kettle and burn his hands. They had to be bandaged and because he was now unable to play with his highchair toys (or the spoons and food), he wouldn't eat anything without a distraction. In desperation Tanya resorted to the TV. I encouraged her to wean him off this habit as soon as possible, as the longer it continued, the harder it would be to change. Without television, Harry fussed and lost interest in his meals for a day or two. But Tanya and Ivan remained firm, and within 48 hours Harry was able to eat a meal without the distraction.

By this time, Tanya had been in contact with me for almost two months. She had already had a good four months of feeding (solids) issues with Harry, not to mention the months of reflux earlier on. She had begun to feel as if her whole life was revolving around her son's feeding, and that she was making slow progress. I continued to emphasise that Harry needed time to adapt to textures. However, Tanya became increasingly stressed by the fact that although Harry had put on some weight, he was still underweight for his age (at the lower end of the centile charts), and that, compared to other toddlers of his age, he didn't eat much.

As a result of the TV dependence and the burns to his hands, Harry's appetite had diminished. Tanya had a couple of miserable weeks and then contacted me again. At this point I had to encourage her to take a step back and look at the facts:

* Harry was genetically slim. Both Tanya and Ivan had been skinny children, and Harry would always have a light frame. His weight compared to other children was not a concern, providing he was eating a sensible, healthy diet.

* Harry was a very active little boy who burned calories quickly. He would not starve. Toddlers will eat when they are hungry, providing their appetites haven't been ruined by excessive snacking.

I also wanted to encourage Tanya to feel less anxious. Being relaxed seemed to give her more confidence when feeding Harry.

With this new confidence we started on part two of the strategy: progression to textured food. Again we revisited Harry's feeding routine and made four key amendments: having his morning milk and breakfast earlier (to be finished by 7.10am and 7.50am respectively); only giving him yoghurt and fruit for breakfast instead of porridge; adding more textures to the puréed foods he enjoyed at lunchtime (i.e. peas, bits of chicken, couscous); and dropping his afternoon milk completely. It took a little while for this strategy to work. Harry wasn't convinced, but I advised Tanya to give him porridge if he didn't eat his lunch in order to give him some carbohydrates to sustain him. I also encouraged Tanya to remain firm when he wouldn't eat. Slowly Tanya's patience and confidence increased, particularly when, within a couple of days, Harry was trying a few more textures than before.

Then Harry started waking earlier in the mornings in a very grumpy mood. Tanya would normally be able to leave him chatting in his cot until just before 7am, even if he woke at 6am, but not any more. He woke any time from 5.15am, and by 6am would be screaming the house down. He would then guzzle his milk and cry for more when he'd finished his bottle. I concluded that he wasn't getting enough food to sustain him through the night, and suggested Tanya give him baby rice with a small amount of fruit after his tea to boost his carbohydrate intake. I also recommended that she cut his morning nap from 45 to 20 minutes, but increase his lunchtime nap from 1 hour and 20–30 minutes to 1 hour and 40 minutes. Again, patience was important. It wouldn't happen overnight as his system needed to adapt to the changes. After three days, Harry suddenly seemed to click back into his normal sleeping habits; in fact he started sleeping even later (until around 7am), which was previously unheard of.

Three months later and Harry has made huge progress. He is now happy with more textured food and will try most finger foods. Tanya feels he's well on the road to eating 'grown-up' food.

Case Studies

Refusing to Feed Himself

Ben – four years

Ben was soon to have his lunch at nursery, but the nursery had made it clear they would not have time to spoon-feed him. Ben had had problems with slow weight gain, and his mother, Susan, had always helped him to eat. While he would eat yoghurt and ice cream with a spoon, he refused to feed himself any other foods. In desperation, Susan contacted me. I gave her the following advice:

* There would be no more spoon-feeding!
* Susan should check Ben's fluid intake by measuring out juice and water at the start of the day, to ensure he got the right balance of fluids, but at the right times and not so much that it affected his appetite.
* Drinks should only be offered after he had eaten most of his meal, and midway between meals.
* Ben was having a very large breakfast and I advised that this amount of cereal should be reduced by half, and replaced with fruit so that he was hungry for lunch.
* Susan should not overload his plate with too much food.
* She should not make a big fuss if Ben used his fingers rather than his spoon or fork.
* She should eat with Ben, even if it was just a mini-version of his meal.
* He would not be forced to eat. If he refused, Susan should say, 'That's fine', and take the plate away.

The first day I suggested Susan put one small broccoli floret, three slices of carrot, and one small diced potato on Ben's plate and ask him to eat them while the chicken nuggets were cooking. He ate these with his fingers with no fuss, then had one nugget and a further small serving of vegetables, followed by another chicken nugget. He went on to eat a fromage frais and some fruit, using his spoon.

Over the following week, Susan followed the same pattern of offering Ben small amounts of vegetables and carbohydrates, while cooking the chicken or fish fingers, which were then offered before giving him more vegetables. Once she had cooked the fish fingers or chicken, Susan sat down with Ben and ate the same food. At this stage it didn't matter if his meals were repetitive; the important thing was that he was offered food he liked and that he was eating it by himself. Some days he would refuse to eat after only a few mouthfuls, and would ask Susan to feed him. When this happened, she would simply remove his plate without making a fuss, but he would not be given the fromage frais and fruit.

During the second week I suggested that Susan invite one of Ben's friends to lunch, and that she buy two sets of special children's cutlery with matching plates. Susan decided to cook chicken casserole, and I advised her to offer both boys a small portion and to explain that once they had eaten it they could have more. If Ben attempted to eat the meal with his fingers, Susan was not to comment upon it. Instead she should say how clever Tom was at using the special cutlery.

On the day, Tom finished his portion within a few minutes, and Susan gave him lots of praise. Ben was still fussing and playing with his food by the time Tom had finished his second portion, but Susan ignored this and offered Tom ice cream and strawberries. Ben immediately kicked up a fuss, demanding the same. Susan was firm and said strawberries and ice cream were for big boys like Tom who ate with his spoon and fork, and that once he had finished he could have strawberries and ice cream. Although Ben did fuss and grumble, he managed to finish his food. Because this was the first time he had used a spoon and fork to eat his meal, Susan did not push him to have a second portion. Instead she gave him lots of praise for using his spoon and fork like a big boy, and allowed him the dessert.

Over the weeks, Susan continued to serve Ben food that he had to eat with a spoon and fork – risottos, spaghetti Bolognese and casseroles, etc. She gradually increased the amount on his plate until he was getting a full portion. If he happily ate two-thirds of the meal, he would get pudding. However, if he fussed and refused to eat, she would silently remove the plate and take him away from the table.

It is very important to allow children of Ben's age control over what they eat, and not to cajole or force them when they appear to eat less. It is fine to offer a pudding or a treat at mealtimes if they have eaten well, but avoid saying, 'If you eat your savoury, you can have an ice cream.' Instead, say, 'When we have finished our savoury we can have some ice cream', which is a more positive statement. If a child refuses the first course, do not get into discussions about treats. Simply remove him from the table and don't mention food until the next snack or meal.

Although it was difficult at times, Susan stuck rigidly to my advice and within a month Ben was happily feeding himself and eating a healthy and varied diet.

Questions and Answers

Q: I am having a testing time with my 17-month-old daughter. She is fast changing from a terrific eater to a real fusspot. She will eat brilliantly at nursery – sometimes even having seconds! – yet at home she always pushes the spoon away. She likes feeding herself, but when I get in from work I just want something quick and easy, otherwise it gets too late and she becomes tired and irritable.

A: Don't worry too much if your daughter is not hungry after nursery. It sounds as if she eats very well while there during the day, possibly because it's more like a fun game to eat with other children. While adults often eat from habit, even if we're not hungry, young children naturally tend to regulate their intake to match their calorie requirements more closely. Thus, if your daughter has eaten a lot earlier in the day, she may not have a great appetite at night. Getting food on the table quickly can help matters at this time of day, though. As you mention, children can get tired and grumpy in the evening, and this can make them less likely to sit and eat. If your daughter has already had a cooked meal at nursery, you could try tempting her with soup and toast (especially in the colder weather) or a simple sandwich. If she needs something more substantial, here are a few quick and easy meal ideas:

* pasta with a commercial tomato pasta sauce (check for those with little or no salt added) and grated cheese
* pasta or rice with a spoon of cream cheese, protein food such as chopped chicken or tinned salmon, and vegetables such as chopped tomatoes, tinned sweetcorn (without added salt) or frozen peas
* pitta bread wrapped around tinned tuna, chopped tomatoes and a little cheese, maybe warmed in the oven or microwave
* baked potato (cooked in the microwave if time is short) with beans or tuna mayonnaise, and carrot and celery sticks on the side
* scrambled egg with finely sliced red and green peppers, served with toast fingers

The amount toddlers eat in a day can vary widely, but at your daughter's age her diet would, as a rule, comprise three small meals and two snacks daily, including three or four portions of carbohydrate or starchy foods (bread, other grain foods and potatoes), five portions of fruit and vegetables, two portions of meat and meat alternatives, and up to 510 ml (17 oz) – minimum of 360 ml (12 oz) – full fat milk per day (or equivalent dairy foods). Do note that many energetic children will eat more than this, and that appetites go up and down. Therefore, don't be concerned if your daughter's intake doesn't match these guidelines every day; think of it as an average intake over three or four days. Your health visitor or GP will be able to check her progress if you have any concerns. However, you can be reassured that your daughter's weight and height are well within normal ranges, with her height a little over the 91st centile and her weight at about the 50th centile.

Q: My little girl will turn two next month. Over the past few weeks I've been getting concerned that she's not eating enough. She used to guzzle every meal, no matter what was offered, but now she just picks at some meals and I can't seem to do anything to make her finish what's on the plate.

A: Just as you can lead a horse to water but can't make it drink, there is sometimes nothing you can do to get your toddler to eat a meal. But this is generally no cause for concern. Virtually every child naturally eats enough to satisfy their needs, but it is often not spread evenly between the three meals of each day. They may pick at breakfast and lunch, and then demolish several platefuls in the evening. Or they may eat like a sparrow for a full day but make up for it with super-sized portions the next day. To reassure yourself you could keep a three-day food diary to examine your child's feeding patterns. Add up how many portions she has eaten from each food group: dairy; meat, fish, poultry and alternatives; fruit and vegetables; and carbohydrates or starchy foods. Divide this by three to get an average amount per day and then look at your daughter's overall intake. Another tip is to check that your daughter isn't drinking more than the recommended amount of milk, or any more than small amounts of sweetened drinks (including fruit juices), as these can affect a child's appetite for solid foods, especially if given just prior to meals. If you need extra reassurance you could get your health visitor or GP to check her height and weight.

You may wonder why your growing daughter seems to be eating less, yet remains quite healthy. Children naturally reduce their food intake relative to their body weight as they age (in other words, they need fewer calories per kilogram of body weight), and this is most obvious during a child's second year. This happens because a baby's rate of growth is most rapid during their first year – they approximately triple their weight during this time. This slows dramatically to about a 25 per cent weight increase during their second year.

Q: My daughter of 15 months will not eat meat. I have tried to disguise it by mincing and adding it to dishes. Since we moved house a month ago, she is refusing most foods and only accepting those she likes and knows. Previously she was an excellent feeder. I now can only get her to eat bread, rusks, cereal, lentil soup and apple. At present she takes 210 ml (7 oz) of milk at 7.15am followed by five or six tablespoons of muesli or Readybrek mixed with chopped fruit and 90 ml (3 oz) of milk, as well as a dozen dry Shreddies and two mini rice cakes. She is offered well-diluted juice throughout the day. Lunch at 11.50am is a slice of cucumber, a piece of brown bread, an apple and a biscuit toast. She takes 120 ml (4 oz) of milk at 3pm. Tea at 5pm is lentil soup, a rusk and a yoghurt. She has a further 180 ml (6 oz) of milk before bedtime.

A: Your daughter is at an age where fussy eating can become a problem. After the first year a baby's appetite does decrease quite a lot and it can be worrying when a baby refuses foods that were previously accepted. Try keeping a food diary as this will help you look at her food intake over the period of a week rather than day by day. If you see the full picture you may find that, apart from her unwillingness to take in meat, she is eating a balanced if somewhat limited diet.

Cutting back on breakfast is a good idea. Begin to offer her milk from a cup at breakfast rather than having a 210 ml (7 oz) feed before the meal. Offer her natural yoghurt mixed with cut or grated fruit, and a few finger foods. When dealing with a fussy eater it is easy to keep offering food throughout the day in an attempt to make her eat something. However, stay with three meals a day until she appears happier to eat a wider variety of food. Only offer her a snack midway between meals if she really seems hungry, and limit snacks to fruit rather than breadsticks or bread, which may fill her up too much before her next meal. Watch her fluid intake, which could also be knocking the edge off an already small appetite, and only offer her a drink of water midway between meals. Remove her cup once she has had a drink, rather than leaving it in sight where she may sip on it throughout the day.

By the age of one year a baby needs a daily minimum of 360 ml (12 oz) of milk (or equivalent other dairy foods), including milk used on cereals and in cooking. Cut out the 3pm feed and replace it with water. This should help increase her appetite for tea. If you stop offering her cereal at breakfast, give her a small bowl of cereal after her savoury tea so you know that she has had enough carbohydrates to see her through the night.

Once you have cut back on her breakfast you may also find your daughter more willing to try something different at lunch. As she likes bread and rusks, try spreading them with puréed casserole. Begin with a very small amount and gradually increase it so she gets used to the taste. It can take time to get a baby interested in food again. Keep using finger foods and offer them with dips such as thick cheese sauce. Lentils are a form of protein so your daughter is receiving a small amount if she continues to enjoy the lentil soup, and you may be able to enrich it by adding a very small amount of grated cheese. Make sure the food you are offering her looks attractive, as this may encourage her to try different things. Giving her small amounts of several different foods, laid out in an eye-catching way, could appeal more than one or two foods mixed together.

Try to eat at least one meal a day with your daughter as she may be encouraged to eat more if she sees you enjoying the same meal. You are right to keep mealtimes happy, as a baby will quickly pick up on any tension you may be feeling about her small appetite. Make mealtimes short and just remove any uneaten food once it is obvious your daughter has finished. If, despite your continuing efforts, she still seems to reject most forms of meat, discuss your concerns with your health visitor or doctor.

Q: My 18-month-old son eats quite well, and drinks water and milk. I try to feed him all the healthiest food, as I know how important it is. I've seen advertisements for various toddler milks and wonder if I should be giving him these rather than regular cows' milk?

A: 'Toddler milks' are marketed as being nutritionally superior to cows' milk, and it is true that they contain a wider range of nutrients such as vitamins and minerals, particularly iron. However, this does not mean that they are a necessity. Younger babies need breast milk or a formula that meets all of their nutritional requirements, including vitamins and protein, because they are not getting any – or much – other nutrition from solids. Beyond the age of one, however, children usually get the vast majority of their nutrition from solids. So long as they generally eat the recommended amounts from each of the food groups and are growing normally, the only nutrients most will require from milk are those found in cows' milk and other dairy foods, including protein, calcium and vitamin B2. Some toddler milks also contain added sugar, which cows' milk does not. While this will certainly encourage a child to drink the toddler milk, it could potentially lead to a taste for sweet drinks.

There may be a place for toddler milk or follow-on formulas for children who are fussy eaters, have a very poor appetite, or are not growing at the usual rate, but it sounds as though your son is eating well. Parents who are concerned about their child's diet could consult *The Contented Child's Food Bible*, published by Vermilion, for more guidance, particularly on iron-rich foods. Do bear in mind that toddler milks are a lot more expensive than cows' milk, and simply offering cows' milk with a daily multi-vitamin and mineral supplement may be a suitable and cheaper alternative. I'd recommend that parents who feel there may be a problem with their child's growth or food intake discuss this, and the use of supplements or toddler milks for children over the age of one, with their GP or health visitor.

Q: My seven-year-old son does seem to eat the right amounts of fruit and vegetables, but it's almost always peas, corn, apples and a bit of orange juice. Is this good enough?

A: Congratulations on having a son who meets his fruit and vegetable requirements at an age when so many children don't. You're correct, though, that this is not always enough to get the best nutrition – variety is key. As a rule of thumb, we should all try to eat a few different colours of vegetables and several different types of fruit each day to get as wide a range of nutrients as possible. Your child is doing well here, with green peas and yellow corn, and the apples and orange juice make up the two different types of fruit. Together these provide fibre, some carbohydrate (starch from these particular vegetables, as well as fruit sugars) for energy, and a host of vitamins, notably vitamin C and folate from the orange juice, and vitamin B1 (required for the body to convert carbohydrates into energy, and for a healthy nervous system) from the peas. (See page 73 for more on this.)

While your son is eating the recommended two types of fruit and vegetables each day, it would be even better if he could increase the variety of fruit and vegetables he enjoys, to further expand the range of nutrients he takes in from this food group. Also, there's always a chance that he may get bored with his current favourites. As a first step to increasing variety you could try different types of fruit juice, though do note that it's best to limit juice to 150 ml (5 oz) of pure fruit juice daily, preferably diluted with water to make it go further. Whole oranges or other citrus fruit would also be a better choice than juice as they contain more fibre. And don't forget that while juice is one alternative to fresh fruit, fruit can also be eaten tinned (preferably in juice) or dried, and you can buy frozen fruit from larger supermarkets as another convenient alternative. Frozen vegetables are also handy to have in the freezer, along with canned vegetables (preferably without added salt) in the pantry.

For a different approach, try taking your son to the supermarket or greengrocer to choose a fruit or vegetable he has never seen before. If he can help you to prepare or cook this food it will probably make him even keener to try it. He might also enjoy growing a few vegetables from seeds if you have the space. Beans and carrots are easy ones to start with. (See page 21 for more ideas on how to make fruit and vegetables tempting to young palates.)

Q: My partner and I are both watching our weight and eating low-fat foods and artificially sweetened foods and drinks. Are these safe to give to my six-year-old son to save me buying two of each product?

A: It can be confusing to combine a healthy low-fat diet for adults with a nutritious diet for children, which contains plenty of foods often shunned by dieting parents, such as full-fat milk or cheese. As children reach the age of five, however, they can complete their transition to an adult-type diet that fits in with family life. For example, after drinking full-fat cows' milk from the age of one to two, children can then change to semi-skimmed milk. From the age of five they can have skimmed milk and reduced-fat dairy products if they are growing well. This change occurs because babies and younger children require higher amounts of fat from food, and more of a group of vitamins that are absorbed into the body with this fat, for healthy growth. As children get older, their growth rate slows and their fat and vitamin requirements are lower, relative to their body weight.

After they turn five children can also eat other low-fat or reduced-fat foods, such as biscuits or ready meals. Do note that many of these foods (for example, crisps and sugary desserts) are best limited to occasional items in the diets of both children and adults. Other foods, such as reduced-fat yoghurts or cheeses, however, can be everyday items. Do also be aware that some reduced-fat foods, such as biscuits, can be higher in sugar than the regular types.

Just as there are a huge number of reduced-fat products in the supermarket, artificial sweeteners are being added to an increasing range of foods, from squashes to mineral waters to yoghurts. The concern is that, if parents are not vigilant, children might consume these sweeteners in many different foods and drinks they eat. My suggestion is to keep any consumption of artificial sweeteners to a minimum, and to check the labels.

If you are giving drinks or other foods containing artificial sweeteners to children, try to vary the type of sweetener. This reduces the risk of consuming too much of any one type. There is a guideline from the British Food Standards Agency recommending not more than three cups – of about 180 ml (6 fl oz) each – a day of squash containing cyclamate for children aged between one and four-and-a-half. And for children under the age of four, be sure to dilute artificially sweetened drinks more than you usually would, to minimise the amount of sweetener. Better still, stick to water and milk as the main drinks, maybe with a little pure fruit juice. Children will be less likely to develop a sweet tooth if they do not have sweet drinks as their usual thirst-quenchers.

Q: I offer my four-year-old son a treat for particularly good behaviour, or in difficult situations such as when I have to make an important phone call. I'm trying not to let him have too many, but wondered how often is too often and what foods would be best to offer?

A: That's a good question, because it is easy to get into the habit of giving a lot of treats. The point of a treat is that it is an out-of-the-ordinary, special occurrence. This means that if they are given too often – once or more each day, for example – they will just become part of the regular diet and will cease to be special. This can bring two problems. Firstly, the diet will not be as healthy if the treat is a food that should only be eaten occasionally. The other issue is that parents may then have to find other treats that are more special to reward (or entice) particularly good behaviour. Thus I'd suggest trying to limit treats to not more than two or three times a week, so they remain special. I do know that this may be difficult – many children are very good at using 'pester-power' to achieve as many treats as possible.

If a treat is only given occasionally it doesn't matter too much if it is not a very healthy food. Just be sure to limit the amount, remembering that children eat a smaller diet than adults and only need a child-sized portion of a treat food. For example, offer one or two chocolate buttons or a mini-chocolate bar rather than a regular-sized one. However, there are many healthy foods that are a special treat to children, especially the younger ones. Here are a few suggestions:

* dried fruit, such as apples, apricots and peaches, cut into star, moon and circle shapes
* a meal placed on the plate to look like a face, or a shape such as a sailing ship on bread as an open sandwich (using cheese or meat slices, cherry tomatoes, cucumber, etc.)
* a strawberry smoothie, placing a strawberry on the rim of the cup for a child-friendly cocktail
* mini-portions of cheese, such as Babybels
* fruit served as a kebab on a wooden skewer (for children who are old enough)
* child-sized yoghurt or fromage frais pots decorated with television characters

To find 'handbag treats' for emergency situations when you are out, have a look at the children's food section in a supermarket. You will find myriad fruit bars, dried fruit packs and muesli bars. If you usually stick to fresh fruit, breadsticks and other plain snacks, your child will view his own, brightly-coloured pack of dried fruit pieces or a muesli bar as an exciting treat. You, meanwhile, will feel safe in the knowledge that the treat is a great source of vitamins, minerals and fibre, though it may contain more sugar than foods you usually choose.

One final suggestion: a small star-shaped sticker is generally a very popular reward for younger children. You will have no concerns about nutrition, and a sheet of stickers fits well in any handbag. Remember also that children do respond well to praise for good behaviour, and this will increase the likelihood they will behave (without the promise of treats) the next time.

Q: My three-year-old has developed a real sweet tooth, and often refuses her main course, only eating pudding. She also prefers sweet snacks and juice between meals. How can I make sure she's eating a healthy diet and not just sugar?

A: Scientists have found that humans recognise and prefer sweet foods from the first day we are born, so it's not surprising that children can develop a sweet tooth. However, some children elevate this to an art form! The problem with eating a lot of sweet foods is that it can make the diet unbalanced – children fill up with the sugary foods (which are often lower in vitamins, protein and other nutrients) so they can't eat enough of the foods their bodies do require. I'd suggest two changes: making the sweet options as healthy as possible, and also encouraging more savoury foods (which I'm sure you're already doing).

As sugar is a natural substance, it can be found in healthy foods, particularly fruit. Here are some sweet but nutritious snack ideas:

* plain fromage frais or cream cheese mixed with fruit purée as a dip for breadsticks or plain crackers
* dried or fresh fruit
* smoothie made with milk and/or yoghurt and fruit such as bananas, peaches canned in juice, or berries
* peanut butter and banana sandwich (if there is no history of nut allergies)
* a container of apple chunks and cubes of cheese
* natural yoghurt mixed with fruit purée and topped with crunchy muesli or other breakfast cereal

Fruit flavours also go well with many savoury foods and can be a great way to add sweetness and encourage children to eat protein-rich foods such as meat. For children over a year honey works well, too, particularly with poultry and pork.

Don't forget that some vegetables, including carrots and corn, contain natural sugars and can add a little sweetness to savoury foods. For example:

* Add grated apple, along with grated carrot and courgette, to homemade meatballs or burgers.
* Toss in sultanas when cooking couscous, then add chopped pineapple and any vegetables your daughter enjoys.
* If stir frying chicken, pork or Quorn, or cooking salmon, squeeze in fresh orange juice (or lemon juice), and drizzle in some honey when it's almost cooked.
* Add chopped apple and apricot to vegetables when cooking lentils or making nut-loaf.
* Bake chicken legs (fun for children to pick up and eat) with apricots tinned in juice and a sprinkle of mild spices such as cumin and coriander.
* Grill kebabs made of meat, poultry, firm tofu or tempeh chunks interspersed with chunks of fruit such as tinned pineapple and fresh peach. You could also add peppers and cherry tomatoes. Be sure the skewers used are blunt and that your child is supervised while eating from them.

To encourage your child to try more savoury foods, the first step is to offer them when she's hungry. Try decreasing the size of between-meal snacks to ensure your daughter is really looking forward to her meals, and offer water rather than juice between meals to quench thirst. If she refuses water, gradually dilute the juice more and more until it is only about one-fifth pure juice to four-fifths water. Then, at the main meal, offer savoury foods to your daughter while eating the same foods yourself and obviously enjoying them. Let your daughter know that she can just take a small taste of each food, and that she can spit it out if she doesn't like it. Give her lots of praise when she eats any of it. Do not offer any dessert until you have finished the main course, and then only one child-sized portion. As she gets used to eating her main meals, gradually decrease the fruit added until she is eating regular savoury foods again.

Q: My daughter is mad keen on cheese. For the past six months, since she turned five, she would happily eat it three meals a day, though I do encourage other foods. I know adults shouldn't eat too much cheese because of the fat content, but is it okay for my daughter to eat it every day, and should I be buying some types and not others? She quite likes Camembert, but is this a problem for children as it is for pregnant women?

A: Cheese is a very nutritious food, packed with muscle-building protein, and important vitamins and minerals. These include calcium, essential for growing bones and teeth, as well as vitamins A, B12 and D (which is required for calcium absorption). Cheese generally contains about 20–40 per cent fat, which is high; however, it's still a valuable food for children as it contains so many other nutrients. On the other hand, if you wanted to buy reduced-fat cheese for the rest of the family for health reasons, your daughter and other children over the age of five can enjoy it too.

When choosing cheese for children, I would suggest that you take note of the salt and calcium content, particularly as your daughter obviously enjoys cheese often. Cheeses vary markedly in their salt content. (On the label you will usually see the salt content listed as sodium, a chemical found in salt, which has the scientific name sodium chloride. See page 56 for more on this.) Salt is added during the making of cheese for a number of reasons, to add flavour and act as a preservative, for example. Lower salt cheeses include cottage cheese and cream cheeses. Brie, Camembert and Cheddar contain higher amounts, Gouda and Edam have a higher salt content still, and processed cheese slices and feta cheese are in the highest salt group. While cheese doesn't ever fit the British Food Standards Agency's guidelines for foods low in salt (0.3 g salt or 0.1 g sodium per 100 g, or less), we can help to minimise our children's salt intake by choosing varieties that are lower in salt most of the time.

Calcium content also varies between types of cheese. It is particularly low in soft fresh cheeses such as cottage cheese, ricotta and cream cheese, which is a shame because, as mentioned above, they are lower in salt. Stilton, feta and Camembert are also lower in calcium than most other cheeses, though they still contain valuable amounts. Other cheeses, such as Cheddar and Edam, are generally very good sources of calcium, while Parmesan is particularly high. Choosing a dairy food such as cheese brings the added advantage of better calcium absorption, thought to be due to the lactose or milk sugar found in dairy products. And there's another bonus: scientists have found that eating cheese at the end of a meal can protect against tooth decay.

If your daughter likes cheese, it's fine for her to eat it every day. This includes Camembert and others not recommended during pregnancy (though they shouldn't be given to babies less than a year old). Brie and Cheddar would be better regular choices than Camembert, though, in terms of calcium content, while containing a similar amount of salt. The amount of cheese she could eat depends on how much other dairy she eats (milk and yoghurt). At five years of age, the recommended minimum amount of dairy foods is 360 ml (12 oz) of milk, or the equivalent amount of other dairy foods, each day. (This is the recommendation from the age of two; between the ages of one and two, it is 360–510 ml (12–17 oz)). A 30 g (1 oz) portion of cheese (about the size of a matchbox) is equivalent to 210 ml (7 oz) of milk, so just two such servings will be enough to meet your daughter's dairy requirement each day. If she is eating much more than the recommended amount, check that she is not eating so much dairy food that she is too full to eat recommended amounts from other food groups.

Useful Addresses

General
Allergy in Schools
www.allergyinschools.org.uk

Allergy UK
www.allergyuk.org
Helpline: 01322 619898

Anaphylaxis Campaign
www.anaphylaxis.org.uk
Helpline: 01252 542029

British Nutrition Foundation
www.nutrition.org.uk
020 7404 6504

Coeliac UK
www.coeliac.co.uk
Helpline 0870 444 8804

Consensus Action on Salt and Health
www.actiononsalt.org.uk

Fair Trade
www.fairtrade.org

Farm Shops
www.farmersmarkets.net
0845 45 88 420

www.pickyourown.info
0845 45 88 420

www.farmshop.uk.com
01427 787 076

Fish
Marine Stewardship Council
www.msc.org

Marine Conservation Society
www.fishonline.org

Food Standards Agency
www.food.gov.uk
www.eatwell.gov.uk

Vegetable Box Schemes
Abel and Cole Ltd
www.abelandcole.co.uk
Tel: 08452 62 62 62

The Organic Delivery Company
www.organicdelivery.co.uk
Tel: 0207 739 8181

Riverford Organic Vegetables
www.riverford.co.uk
0845 600 2311

Organic Food
The Soil Association
www.soilassociation.org
Tel: 0117 314 5000

www.soilassociationscotland.org
Tel: 0131 606 2474

Organic Meat
Eastbrooks Farm Organic Meat
www.helenbrowningorganics.co.uk
01739 790340

Sheepdrove Organic Farm
www.sheepdrove.com
01488 674 747

Organic Milk
www.omsco.co.uk
01934 511 115

Vegan Society
www.vegansociety.com
0121 523 1730

Vegetarian Society
www.vegsoc.org
0161 925 2000

Index

abdominal pain 80
additives 53, 55, 58, 61, 162
allergic reaction 36, 82
allergies 13, 32, 40, 55, 64,
    69, 77, 113
    food 79, 81–5, 162
anthocyanidins 72, 73, 74
antibiotics 13, 24, 28, 35, 40
antioxidants 16, 40, 44, 72–4
appetite 79–80, 93, 94, 101

bacon 28
bacteria 30, 36, 45, 78, 156
    beneficial 40, 77
bananas 14, 15, 16, 77, 98
Banana Loaf 225
Banana Muffins 218
barley 46, 47
    Baked Barley Risotto 212
beans 14, 48, 126
    Hearty Bean Soup 180
beef 25–6
    Minced Beef Cobbler 194
    Pot-Roast 202
berries 73, 76, 98, 99
beta-carotene 12, 73
biscuits 52–3, 57, 59, 102
blackcurrants 143
blender 109, 131
bottles 62, 63, 152
bread 47, 52, 58, 76, 149, 160
    making 131–2, 135, 226
breadcrumbs 48, 59, 114
breadmaker 131–2
breakfast 37, 38, 59, 96–100
breakfast cereals 56, 59, 76–7,
    98, 99, 127
brunch 37, 38, 100
bulghar wheat 46, 47, 124
Burger recipes 166, 177
butter 125, 149

cakes 52–3, 57, 59, 156
    Autumn Apple Cake 230
    Banana Loaf 225
    Courgette Cake 229
calcium 34, 35, 39, 40, 41, 46,
    88, 266
carbohydrate 44, 46, 52, 97
carotenoids 72, 73, 74

carrots 11, 15, 16, 73
cereal bars 152
cheese 39, 41, 90, 125, 141,
    263, 265–7
chemicals 12, 13, 14, 40, 58
chicken 12, 14, 24, 28 9, 93
    broth 94
    Crunchy-topped 168
    Fruity 170
    'Hiccup' 172
    Pitta Pockets 178
    nuggets 147
    roast 24, 29, 59
    Sticky Chicken Thighs 165
    and Vegetable Bake 196
    and Vegetable Stir Fry 189
chicken stock 108
chickpeas 43, 44, 49, 126
    in Tomato Sauce 164
children, cooking with 53,
    117, 134–40
cholesterol 29, 35, 43, 46,
    47, 72, 88, 97
colic 79, 84
cookies 134, 156
    Apricot 231
Courgette Rosti Cakes 185
couscous 46, 124
    Tomato and Mint 192
crisps 102, 162
curry 26
    Chicken 'Hiccup' 172
    Salmon and Coconut 190

dairy products 39–42, 52,
    87–8, 93, 267
defrosting food 130
dehydration 92, 107, 156
desserts 105, 141–4, 149, 156,
    223–8
dips 21, 103, 151, 155
    eggy 37–8
    recipes 220–21
    sweet 103, 143
dried fruit 21, 88, 105, 111,
    127, 141, 152, 263
drinks 61 3, 107, 119, 152,
    156, 232

eating out 146–58

Egg-fried Rice 38, 179
eggs 35–8, 73, 81, 83, 88, 125
    breakfasts 99, 100
    freshness test 36
    hard-boiled 37, 154
    omega-3 67
    poached 38, 99
    safety 36
    scrambled 36–7, 99, 100
Eggy Bread 38, 99, 169
essential fatty acids 12, 65
exercise 79

family meals 37, 100, 115–17,
    119, 234
farm shops 11, 35
farmers' markets 11, 27, 35
fat 40, 41, 52, 56, 57, 87
    hydrogenated 56, 57
    low-fat foods 40, 261–2
    meat and poultry 12, 25–9
    polyunsaturated 65
    saturated 47, 56, 88, 90
fibre 16, 43, 44, 47
finger foods 37, 251
first-aid kit, for outings 158
fish 31–4, 52, 83, 93, 147, 236
    Baked with Quinoa 213
    easy meals 69–71
    Fishcakes 176
    Gentle Spiced Monkfish 201
    oily 31, 66, 68–9
    and Prawn Pie 197
    smoked 32, 37, 66
    tinned 34, 124
fish stock 108
flapjacks 46, 151, 156
    Fruity Flapjacks 217
flaxseeds 67, 68
flour 127–8
food intolerance 79, 83–5
food poisoning 29, 32, 36, 45,
    66, 86, 130, 140
food preparation 136–7
food processor 131
food safety 30, 33, 36, 48,
    69, 156–8
free radicals 72
free-range foods 24, 28–9, 35
freezing food 129–30, 235–6

fridge, stocking 125
frittata 37, 154
    Red Pepper and Feta 167
frozen foods 76, 105, 126
vegetables 22, 58, 124, 125
fruit 98, 99, 102, 156, 263
desserts 142, 143, 149
purées 41, 142, 143–4
salad 21, 73, 136, 142, 160
stewed 144
fruit & vegetables 52, 76, 87,
    90, 141, 260–61
    box schemes 10, 17
five-a-day 20, 47, 62
growing your own 14, 113
preparing 14, 22
seasonal 18–19, 144
shopping 11, 16–22
snacks 21, 102, 103, 151
fruit juice 21, 62, 93, 98,
    149, 152
    making 105, 132
fun foods 69, 263
fussy eating 53, 118–21, 153,
    251–3, 256–9

gammon 27
germs 75, 78
gluten 28, 46
Glycaemic Index (GI) 77
GM foods 13, 40
grains 43–7, 52, 93, 124, 126
Guacamole 221

ham 27
healthy diet 52–6, 87–8, 115
herbs 17, 22, 109
highchairs 146
honey 70, 76, 128
hormones 13, 24, 28, 35
hummus 103, 151
Red Pepper 220

ice cream 15, 21, 36, 76, 143
    Strawberry Yoghurt 224
ice lollies 21, 105, 107, 142
illness 80, 92–4
immune system 13, 40, 74,
    75–8, 80, 92
iodine 31, 35, 69
iron 22, 28, 35, 50, 62, 72,
    88, 120, 260

jam 76
jelly 21
journeys 150–52
juicer 132

kitchen equipment 131–2
knives 132, 136, 137

labels 13, 54–6, 90
lactose intolerance 84
lamb 26–7
    Burgers 166
Fillets, with Couscous 192
    Moroccan Lamb 193
    Pot-Roast Herby Lamb 204
Lasagne recipes 198, 200
learning about food 11, 23, 138
Lemonade, Old-fashioned 232
lentils 48, 49, 73, 126
liquidiser 131
liver 29
lunchboxes 21, 37, 73, 159–62
lutein 72, 73, 74
lycopene 72, 73, 74, 124

Macaroni Cheese 207
mackerel 37, 66, 70
Marmite 151
meal planners 234
meat 14, 23–30, 52, 87, 89
Meatballs 166
melons 156
menus 159–60, 238–45
mercury 33, 69
milk 15, 24, 39–40, 52, 63,
    68, 100, 125, 262
    intolerance 81, 83, 84
    toddler milks 259–60
millet 46, 47
mineral water 148
minerals 12, 16, 22, 31, 32,
    35, 40, 52
mouth ulcers 80
muesli 59, 97, 99
muffins 47, 59, 76, 99, 151
    Banana 218
    Carrot and Pear Honey 227
    Courgette Cornmeal 216
    homemade 106, 160
mustard and cress 113

nitrate 66
noodles 126

nursing mother 14, 37, 103
nutrients 52, 53, 87–8
nuts 52, 67, 70, 76, 81, 83,
    87–8, 103, 105, 113

oatcakes 79, 101, 107, 151
    recipe 222
oats 46, 59, 77, 97, 127
oils 56, 67, 70, 128
olives 113
omega-3 fats 56, 64–70
    in fish 31, 34, 66
    non-fish 12, 24, 40, 67
    supplements 69
omega-6 fats 40, 69–70
omelettes 37, 76, 148
organic food 12–15, 24, 27,
    28–9, 31, 35, 39–40
overtiredness 80

pancakes 38, 100, 141, 143
    Oaty 215
parsley 22
pasta 58, 76, 124, 126, 148
    Green Monster 173
    Linguine with Tuna 188
    Salmon and Broccoli 214
sauces 21, 48, 76, 149
    Tagliatelle with Sauce 191
pastry 59
peanut butter 162
pesticides 12, 14, 15, 24, 40
Pesto, Homemade 184
picnics 37, 73, 153–7
pizza 135–6, 148, 154, 182–3
pork 27–8
    Asian Pork Casserole 210
porridge 46, 59, 77, 93, 97
    making 98
portion sizes 20, 79, 119
potatoes 16, 52, 148
    Courgette Rosti Cakes 185

poultry 28–9, 52
prawns 32
    Prawn Risotto 211
prebiotics 77–8
pregnancy 14, 36, 64
preservatives 12, 27, 47
probiotics 68, 77–8
processed foods 52, 53, 55–60,
    70, 90, 93, 147, 162
protein 23, 31, 35, 39, 44,

46, 47, 52, 88, 258–9
puddings 141, 142
    Apple and Date Sponge 228
Chocolate Pudding 223
pulses 21, 43–4, 47–50, 52,
    87–8, 111, 126
purées 70, 76, 108, 131, 141
    freezing 129–30
fruit 41, 142, 143–4

quinoa 44, 46, 47, 52, 124
    Baked Fish with 213

rabbit 29–30
raisins 21, 103, 113, 152
ready-meals 52, 57, 90
refined foods 76–7
reflux 79, 251
refusing food 87, 121, 248–50
reheating food 130, 235
restaurants 146–50
rice 44, 45, 52, 76, 126
    basmati, cooking 45
    Vegetarian 206
risotto 45, 46, 59, 148, 235
    Baked Barley 212
    Prawn 211
Rye Sticks 219

safety, kitchen 140
salad 14, 21, 111–14, 125,
    136, 151, 160
Salad Niçoise 208
    toppings 112–13
salad dressings 112, 128
salmon 32, 66, 70, 71
    and Coconut Curry 190
    Pasta with 214
    smoked 37, 100
    tinned 34, 68, 124
salmonella 29, 36
salt 28, 41, 54, 56, 66, 90,
    149, 151, 266
sandwiches 21, 41, 70, 71,
    148, 151, 160
Chicken Pitta Pockets 178
    fillings 155
sardines 66, 68, 70, 71
sauces 41, 57, 59, 117, 143
sausages 23, 28, 154
Scotch pancakes 38
seasonal foods 11, 18–19
seeds 70, 87–8, 103, 112–13
selenium 31, 35, 72, 74

self-feeding 254–5
shellfish 32–3, 66, 83
shopping 10–50, 54, 117, 235–6
smoothies 21, 46, 62, 72, 93,
    98, 156, 263
    making 104–5
snacks 10, 21, 52, 79, 101–7,
    119, 151, 264
    recipes 215–22
sorbet 21, 76, 142
soup 22, 48, 73, 76, 93, 148
    Carrot, Lentil and Sweet
Potato 187
chicken broth 94
    Chicken Noodle Soup 181
    Hearty Bean Soup 180

homemade 108–10
    Jungle Soup 171
Sweetcorn Chowder 186
soya 52, 67, 83, 87–8, 129
spirulina 67
steak 25
stir-fries 25, 28, 29
    Chicken and Vegetable 189
stock 22, 108, 129
store cupboard 124–9, 236
strawberries 11, 15, 143, 156
sugar 52, 55, 57, 61, 76, 102,
    128, 141, 264–5
sugar-free drinks 61
supplements 69, 70, 88, 93,
    120, 260
Sweetcorn Chowder 186
sweeteners 41, 61, 262

table manners 116, 150
teething 80
texture of food 251–3
tinned food 58, 124, 126
    fish 34, 66, 68, 124, 126
    pulses 43, 111, 126
    tomatoes 73, 124
tofu 67, 88, 105
tomato: and Bean Dip 221
sauce 164, 182
tinned 73, 124, 126
toxins 13, 14, 40, 48, 72, 124
trace elements 52
treats 52–3, 141-4, 262–4
tuna 34, 66
turkey 29
    Burgers 177
    and Leek Lasagne 198

vegetable stock 108
vegetables 11, 52, 93, 125
    cooking 22
    disguising 76, 108
    frozen 22, 58, 124, 125
    leafy 16, 52, 73, 88
    raw 21, 103, 120
    refusing to eat 121
    Roasted, with Couscous 174
    see also fruit & vegetables
Vegetarian Rice 206
vegetarians 47, 48, 69, 86–91
viruses 74, 75, 78
vitamins 12, 16, 19, 22, 31,
    35, 39, 40, 52, 77, 124
    A 73
    B_{12} 88
    C 22, 50, 62, 72, 74, 88, 93
    E 12, 72, 74

walnuts 67, 68, 103, 113
water 63, 77, 79, 92, 148,
    152, 156
wheat 28, 44, 47, 83, 107
wholegrains 43, 44, 47, 58,
    87–8, 98, 99
wraps 59, 60, 155

yoghurt 40–41, 52, 76, 105,
    125, 263
    adding fruit 41, 98, 99,
    107, 142, 143
live 40, 77–8, 93

zinc 80

Acknowledgements

Several people have provided huge support during the writing of Feeding Made Easy. I would like to thank Registered Dietitian Fiona Hinton, Natural Nutritionist Vardit Kohn, and Family Naturopath Lucinda Miller for their valuable advice and expertise on various aspects of the nutritional needs of children and families. I would especially like to thank my personal editor, Kate Bouverie, whose expertise, enthusiasm and dedication have contributed so very much to the book. Thanks are due to Georgina Nunn and Gayle Wilde for their help with compiling recipes, and to Kate Quarry, Posy Ford, Yamini Franzini and Lucy Bottomley, who also provided great insight and recipes. Special thanks also to the many children who tested all the recipes, particularly Iona, Eleanor, Isabella, Rufus, Josiah, Honor, Tara, Ravi, Arun, Edmund, William, Frieda and Minna.

As always, huge thanks are due to my literary agent, Emma Todd who continues to provide immense support and encouragement, and to all the team at Random House, in particular my publisher Fiona MacIntyre and editor Imogen Fortes, who have both guided me through the process of bringing this book into being.

Finally, this book would not be here were it not for the thousands of families who constantly provide me with inspiration and feedback. This book is for all those parents who are striving to feed their families the most nutritious, tastiest food they can. I hope it helps.

The publishers would like to thank Dr Julia Kenny, Specialist Registrar, Paediatrics.

www.contentedbaby.com
In 2004 Gina launched an exclusive website and magazine on-line for parents following the advice in her books. Each month the website publishes interesting features and FAQ's on all aspects of parenting. Healthy eating, swapping recipe ideas and menu planning is one of the major topics always being discussed on the members forums. More details on how to be part of this supportive and dynamic on-line community check can be found on www.contentedbaby.com